STOP WHI...
AND JUST G...
WITH IT!!!
MY LIFE GROWING UP

By
P Roberts

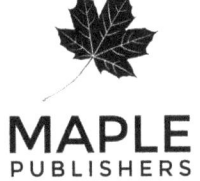

MAPLE
PUBLISHERS

STOP WHINGING AND JUST GET ON WITH IT!!! MY LIFE GROWING UP

Author: P Roberts

Copyright © 2024 P Roberts

The right of P Roberts to be identified as the author of this work has been asserted by the author in accordance with section 77 and 78 of the Copyright, Designs and Patents Act 1988.

ISBN 978-1-83538-463-3 (Paperback)
    978-1-83538-464-0 (Hardback)
    978-1-83538-465-7 (E-Book)

Cover Design and Book Layout by:
    White Magic Studios
    www.whitemagicstudios.co.uk

Published by:
    Maple Publishers
    Fairbourne Drive, Atterbury,
    Milton Keynes,
    MK10 9RG, UK
    www.maplepublishers.com

A CIP catalogue record for this title is available from the British Library.

All rights reserved. No part of this book may be reproduced or translated by any form or by any means, electronic or mechanical, including photocopying, recording or by any information storage and retrieval system without written permission from the author.

The views expressed in this work are solely those of the author and do not necessarily reflect the views of the publisher, and the publisher hereby disclaims any responsibility for them.

After submitting this book in its entirety to my publisher, an unfortunate accident led to me being admitted to Ward 33 at North Tees Hospital with a fractured knee. I wanted to include this to express my gratitude to the staff at all levels for the outstanding care I received during my week-long stay. I believe in giving credit where it's due, and I am sincerely thankful. However, this does not alter the facts or observations presented here.

After our work event on Christmas night, I made my way home during a fierce storm. In my rush to get indoors, I slipped and fell, and the pain was unbearable. Not wanting to trouble anyone, I spent the night on the floor. The next morning, my friend Ann arrived, and we called 999. I now have a full-length plaster cast on my leg.

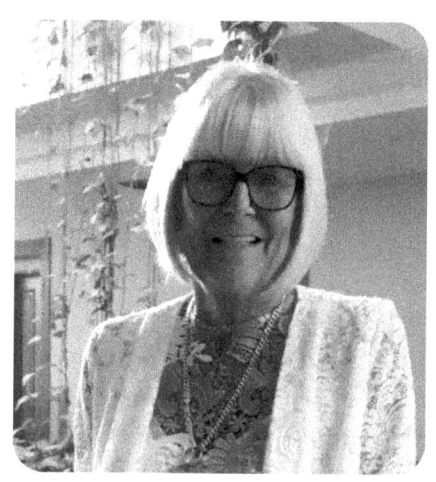

I dedicate this book to Rosie, a truly amazing lady massively missed. RIP

Contents

Hospital 13

Growing up 29

My School Years 58

Working 64

Present Day 83

My furry friends, past and present 97

Hi there, my name is Pauline, I was born on the 20th of January 1953, I am Hartlepool born and bred. You are probably wondering what's behind the title of this book. To some people it may seem a little cheeky, harsh even.

Well, to me it has a double meaning, one - it has been my motto and motivation in life. I contracted Polio when I was 18 months old, affecting my legs. I had two full length callipers to enable me to walk. And because of that, my life has been a constant challenge, overcoming barriers that not everyone has had to face in life, and no, this is not a sympathy vote. I have never let my disability hold me back and I am proud to say I have worked full time all my life. In fact even though I have retired, I still do work on a part time basis and I love it.

One thing that always makes me smile, well the irony of it really, is a certain comment that has been made to me in the past on more than one occasion by various people. They would ask me what my problem was, then after I informed them that I had polio as a baby, their response would be, "Oh well, you've never really known any difference, have you?" Like that makes it alright then. It's the most stupid of comments and could only come from a fit person living a normal life, and I make no apology for using the word 'normal'. Of course I know the difference, being as I'm the one that has had to live with the stigma of it. I will share with you my experiences of this later. Suffice to say, disability was frowned on way back then. Again, this is definitely not a sympathy vote, I'm strong willed and my determination has carried me through.

I have always said, I can do anything you can do. It may be a different way and possibly take a little longer, but I have always been fiercely independent with something to prove and, as the saying goes, necessity is the mother of invention.

The second reason behind the title is, I am 1 of 7 surviving siblings, my mam lost two babies, it was never spoken about so that is all I know. I am the third oldest, Marjorie (Marjy to friends and family) being the oldest then from, oldest to youngest, George, Me, Maureen, (who has now sadly passed) Kevin, Elaine, and Leslie. My mam was called Doreen, (known as Dolly to her family) and my dad was George, (Geordie to his mates). We were brought up on a council estate and we had nothing, none of us on the estate did, and unlike present times there was very little support, available to us, financial or otherwise.

Times were very hard, especially for my mam and dad. Not only did they have seven kids to provide for, but two of them were disabled, me with Polio and my brother George with a quite severe learning disability; this was due to the umbilical cord being round his neck when he was born. But it was pointless whinging about it, **you just had to get on with it**, and as a family, that is exactly what we did. I have always said I would not change my upbringing for the world, I am proud of it. Tough as it was, depravation is an excellent lesson in life, it gives you values and appreciation for the smallest of things, but I certainly would have changed it for my mam and dad. It aged them before their time. My dad was relatively young when he was diagnosed with Parkinson's disease. As I remember he was in his late thirties, it was yet another burden they both had to contend with. Sadly, my mam died when she was just 55 years old. She died of a brain haemorrhage. I had left home by this time as most of us had, the only two of us still living at home, was obviously my brother George, who would never be able to live independently due to the severity of his learning disability, and the youngest of us, my brother Les.

I can still remember the day a call came into my work requesting I go home immediately, 'home' meaning the family abode. A reason was not given but I just knew it had to be serious, I actually thought it was my dad, being as he was the one who had been in ill health for years with his Parkinson's disease, so to find that mam had died like that, so unexpectedly was such a devastating shock to us all. However not half as devastating as it was for my dad and brother George; their lives were about to be turned upside down as both relied heavily on the care my mam gave them, particularly George, as her life revolved around his needs, and he idolised her. Normally mam was first up every morning, fire lit, kettle on etc. Not this time though. In fact, it was my brother George that had found her, but because of his learning disability, he didn't fully understand what had happened. He just rushed downstairs and said to my dad, "Mam's asleep on the bedroom floor, and I can't wake her up." Some memories never leave you, I can still see our George, bless him, looking out of the front window, as they carried her out, crying and asking, "Where they taking me mam?" As I said she had died from a brain haemorrhage. A cruel, tragic end for an absolutely amazing, wonderful mother taken from us far too soon.

Now then, what prompted me to write this book? Well, not only did I want a trip down memory lane for myself, but I also wanted to share all those memories of my growing up, the hard times and the good times, and for people of today, to take note, and to be responsible for their actions, the choices they make and to realise just how lucky they are. In other words, to **Stop whinging and just get on with it.** We live in a welfare state and thankfully there isn't the poverty today that we experienced, but neither is there the pride and respect that was drilled into us, particularly by my dad. He used to say repeatedly, "If you don't have pride, you have nothing, you are a Roberts, hold your head up, you don't owe anybody anything, and there is no one better than you."

His words have always stayed with me, and so I have gone through life believing it to be true, that yes, there is no one better than me, but also, I am no better than anyone else, I have never really been star struck, in the main for me, I see so called celebrities as divas living a privileged life. I say, so called, as with some individuals, just because they have taken part in, for example, a silly reality show, or some other stupid claim to fame, for me, it does not make them a celebrity, it's a joke to class them as such. I am the first person to recognise and appreciate true talent in which ever field of art it sits. I also recognise and respect the hard work, dedication and the passion applied by the individuals that got them where they are today, so richly deserved.

I also greatly admire people who have contributed to society, making a difference, all too often at a personal cost or sacrifice to themselves thus warranting the all too often, unwelcome recognition earned and so rightly given. When I say it's a joke, it's just one area of things that have gone crazy in this country and not necessarily for the good. For example, when did it become acceptable to sit back on benefits rather than work, to have numerous children and expect the state to keep them, where is the pride in that? And how did the ridiculous situation arise where some people are actually better off on benefits than the people working for a living. The very same people who actually pay for their privilege to do that. I used to be an avid watcher of all political programmes, but now due to the ridiculous situation we find ourselves in, I can't bear to watch or listen to any of it, I don't need a constant reminder of how bad things are, or how worse it is going to get. To my shame I now prefer to bury my head in the sand, and yes, in this instance, ignorance is most definitely bliss. These days I would rather watch Angela Lansbury in, Murder She Wrote, or Dennis Waterman in New Tricks, the good old days, no political correctness, and a little light relief.

For me the Great Britain we had is no more. The system is being constantly abused, I hasten to add, not by everyone. This is NOT a criticism of genuine people, as I wish with all my heart the support of today had been there for my mam and dad. So, before any of you, hard done by people get on your high horses and want to shout me down in indignation, I ask that you read this book in its entirety, and I hope you enjoy sharing an insight into our life's experiences. Then I think you will have to agree, there is no comparison to present day living however hard done by some people may feel.

The first home I can remember was a prefab, number 25 Bowness Grove, Hartlepool. The area was known as WAGGA. (Illustrated) as you will see by the photograph, it was not the most picturesque of settings, sitting on the edge of an industrial estate, but hey, you were just grateful for a roof over your head, and this was home. We lived there until I was approx. ten years old.

Sorry, I'm jumping the gun here a little, I'll start from when I contracted Polio as a baby. An epidemic had hit the town in the mid 1950's. For those of you who are fortunate enough to have never heard of it, I will give you a brief description of this cruel virus. Polio or Poliomyelitis is a disabling and life-threatening disease caused by the Polio virus. The virus spreads from person to person and can infect the spinal cord, causing permanent paralysis. There is no cure, but it is preventable with a vaccine. Apparently, it mainly affects children under five. I was eighteen months old. When in later life, I asked my mam what had happened to me, she said, that one minute I was toddling along with a walker, when suddenly I collapsed and that was that. Polio. It was the start of my numerous admissions to Sedgefield General Hospital, and it was always for long-term stays, the minimum being six months the longest eighteen months.

Polio affected my legs. The right being totally paralysed, the left one, very weak. Obviously at that age I can't remember much. What I can remember is sitting in a big cot surrounded by what felt like big iron bars and me looking through them crying, feeling very alone. I learned very quickly not to cry because my mam never came. It wasn't that I was being neglected as I expect the nurses were very busy, and anyway a nurse is no substitute for a mother. As I remember it was such a heart-breaking feeling of abandonment and isolation. To be suddenly taken away from your mam for months on end as a baby, being denied her natural love and affection growing up had a lasting effect on me emotionally. However, eventually it toughens you up and gives you a sense of independence and an instinct for self-survival. I do know as a child, not being used to close contact, I hated to be kissed or cuddled, I still am a little like that. Any emotion I feel is usually suppressed, and although felt, very rarely displayed. I'm not a touchy-feely person at all, unless it is the four-legged furry species. All my family and friends know I am an animal lover through and through, I can't even kill a fly. In fact, generally I much prefer animals to humans. I was the one that took all the waifs and strays home. The times my mam told me, "You're not bringing that in here; don't you think I've enough to feed?" But being an animal lover herself, she always gave in saying, "It can stay tonight but that's it." Well you can guess the rest, yes, they had found their forever home. The only time she put her foot firmly down was when I rescued a hamster from some kid on our estate, they were getting rid of it. Not having a cage, I improvised, we had a glass fronted unit, so when my mam came home from shopping, it was to discover a little hamster running around in the bottom of it lol, it's fair to say she was not best pleased. In the early days, our furniture was tatty at best, I remember the couch and chairs, I was going to say Three Piece suit but that sounds far too elaborate. Anyway, it was black PVC not very hard wearing, I remember the arms were split with the foam poking through, but the funniest thing was, it had screw in legs that were forever falling off, usually when one of us was sitting on it lol.

Well, that's just an introduction and a bit of a profile to start with. I am now going to timeline and categorise the stages of my life growing up. But first, an apology in advance for some of the language I have used, I felt the need to say it just as it was for us way back then, and anyway, I actually think it is rather funny and atmospheric. I hope you do too. However, if you are easily offended, read no further lol.

Hospital

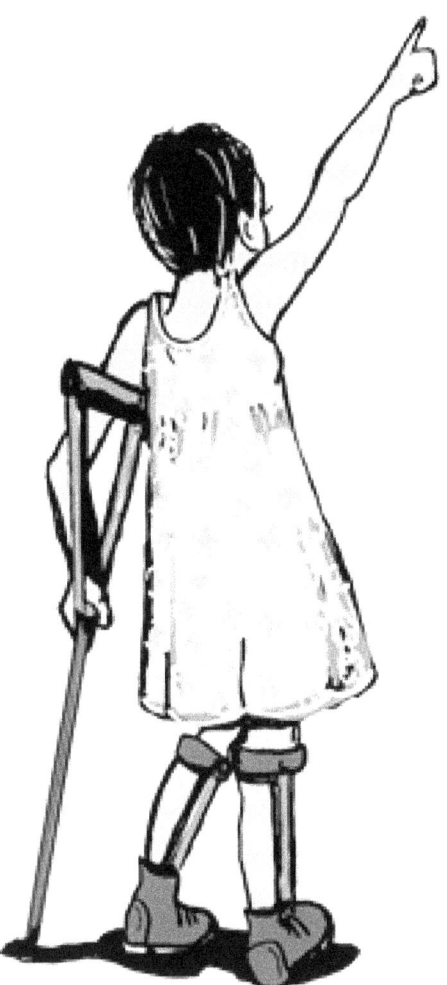

In this section I describe the time I spent in Sedgefield General hospital and how the experience affected my life growing up, from being a baby of eighteen months through to my teenage years. There is also a mention of my time spent as an outpatient at St Hilda's Hospital in Hartlepool.

As I said earlier, it was always a long term stay and always in Sedgefield General Hospital, ward 16, this being the children's ward. It was situated right at the top of a long corridor on the left. I do believe originally the hospital was built to treat injured soldiers of the Second World War, and as I remember the wards were better described as tin huts. I distinctly remember they were of a prefabricated construction, covered in corrugated sheets, they were set out just like an army barracks. Double iron framed glass doors at the side of each ward opened onto a grassy area. All the wards were the same, side by side, and all at ground level. I can also remember big iron heating stoves in the centre of the ward. However, I don't want you to think of this description as me being critical because it couldn't be further from the truth. For a hospital it was truly amazing, the unbelievable homely, friendly atmosphere, the caring staff, and the fact that it was surrounded by countryside. All contributed to a reasonably happy stay.

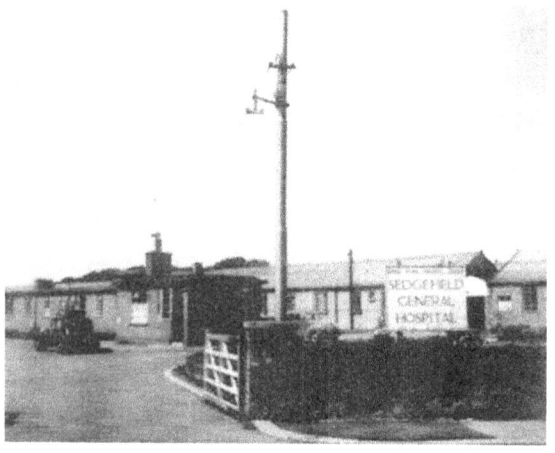

I was in and out of Sedgefield General Hospital for most of my childhood. From being a baby of eighteen months old in the children's ward, then from fifteen or sixteen, in the ladies' ward. Us kids that were long stay, I would say about eight to ten of us, all with various illnesses, were kept separate, you entered our ward through two swing doors at the top of the main ward. It was like our own little community. We had a teacher that used to come and give us lessons for two hours in the afternoon, weekdays. Obviously missing out on that much schooling had to have had an adverse effect on your education. All in all, though I think I came through it quite well.

Sedgefield was a lengthy journey from Hartlepool, cars, obviously were only for the privileged few. Mam relied on buses and because of her other commitments at home and the cost implication, she could only manage to visit me once a week on a Saturday afternoon. I was now past the baby stage and oh, how I looked forward to those visits. The doors would be opened spot on 2pm and not a minute before. The visitors would stream in, and my eyes would never leave them until I saw my mam coming. For all I was overjoyed to see her I still feel guilty to this day that I never let her give me a kiss and a cuddle at the start and end of the visit. It must have hurt her; but I just couldn't connect in that way. It was never intentional and after she left, I always hated myself for it. During the winter months, the snow was so bad the buses couldn't get through, so I wouldn't see my mam for quite a number of weeks. It was such a massive disappointment for me to not see her among the visitors that did manage to make it through. Some of the other kids got visitors nearly every day. I hated those times; I used to pretend I was asleep in case anyone felt sorry for me for not having any visitors. I have despised pity and sympathy all my life and I would get quite indignant if I heard it directed at me. I just hated being singled out and being made to feel different.

Anyway, back to my hospital experiences, I understood even at my young age that my mam could only visit me once a week, I never held it against her. My maternal nana visited me every six weeks or so, and each visit, she would put half a crown (old money) into my piggy bank, it was an amazing treat. I never saw any of my brothers or sisters for the whole time I was in there. Also, it's funny my dad never ever visited me. Again I never gave it a second thought and I didn't hold it against him, I just thought it was the norm. It was later in life he told me he despised the consultant I was under, referring to him as a butcher. Looking back as an adult I am now inclined to agree with him. I won't say his name for obvious reasons, but will refer to him as Mr. X. He was a well-respected Orthopaedic Consultant. Definitely not by my dad though. The numerous operations he did, I feel were experimental at best, and in my opinion did no good whatsoever, in fact I strongly believe they made things worse, particularly to my left leg. It was not paralysed, yet he had it in a calliper for years, that I now believe was not needed, in fact I don't believe my left leg was affected at all, prior to his intervention. It is a proven fact that there is no cure for polio, whatever paralysis it leaves you with is for life. Also, my friends at school, at least five of them, all had the same as me, all victims of Polio and all had callipers on one leg. I used to wonder at the time why not one of them were ever hospitalised or had surgery as I did. They were however under a different consultant to me. It seems I drew the short straw, and I now strongly believe my dad was right. I recently made an online application for my medical records from back then, however I was told they don't keep them from that far back. I don't dwell on this at all, it is what it is and as for my parents consenting to it, well those people in them days were God like in authority and you never questioned them, believing everything they did was for the best. I do remember his name, but again I will refer to him as Mr.

X. I know this may sound heartless, but he did die and as a result I was referred to another consultant, a Mr R Ellis. It was the best thing that happened to me. This guy was amazing, and I have a lot to thank him for. I will expand on my relationship with him later.

The Hospital back then, as I remember, was very much like the TV programme, The Royal, in fact it was exactly like that. Unlike the NHS today, the ward sister was a force to be reckoned with, very well respected and very much in charge, whenever the nurses were asked to do anything, it was, "Yes sister, right away sister, three bags full sister" an element of fear but, mostly respect. Likewise, was the sister's regard and respect towards the Matron and so on through the hierarchy.

Then there were the consultants who came with their entourage, usually once a week they would do their rounds, I can only liken it to a royal visit. Us kids were warned beforehand, not to mess up our beds, all our toys were put away, we just had to sit in our beds on our best behaviour and do nothing until they had completed their rounds and left. I also remember the uniforms, laundered and starched, they were immaculate, as were the wards themselves. Once a week the cleaning ladies would come with their buckets, scrubbing brushes and kneeling pads. They would physically push all of our beds and lockers to one side, then down on hands and knees to scrub every inch of the floor, repeating the same for the other side. I can still smell the disinfectant they used, such hard work. One thing was a certainty, the patient care was first, last and always.

Most of the nurses were absolutely lovely to us. You did get the odd strict, no-nonsense type, and there are a few horrible experiences of which I will reveal later, but in the main they were lovely. During the summer months they would on occasion open the side doors and manually push all our beds outside into the sunshine and fresh air. I mean, how amazing was that? After being confined indoors for months on end, to us this was an unforgettable treat. I have never to this day forgotten the wonderful smell of the great outdoors, it is something that is taken for granted every day without a second thought. We would stay outdoors nearly all day, even having our meals out there, it was like having our own little picnic and we loved every minute of it.

Now, here's a thing, quite shocking really. Have you heard of something called Mercury? It is also known as Quick Silver, liquid metal. Well, it was present in the thermometers, do you get where I'm going with this? No, well I'll tell you, us kids had a little bottle each and we used to collect the Mercury from the broken thermometers. Then we would play with it on our over-bed table. Obviously at the time it can't have been known how toxic it was, or it would never have been allowed. To us it was just a game to see who could get to the broken thermometer first and nab the Mercury. We did on occasion drop them deliberately lol, but we didn't get away with that too often. Anyway, toxic or not we had a lot of fun with it and I'm still here to tell the tale lol.

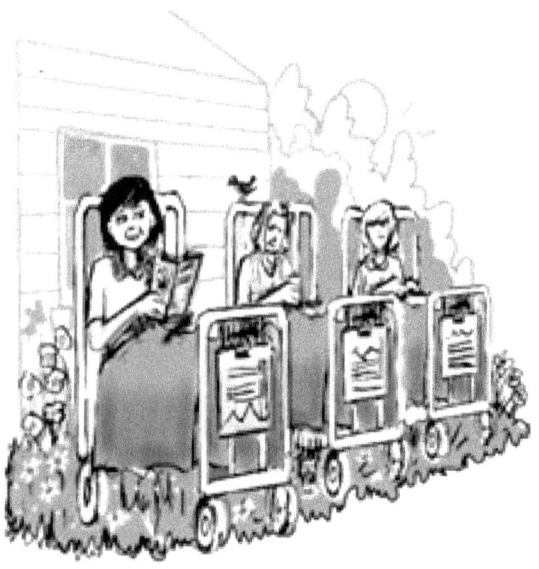

There were lots of happy times, I remember the Christmases I spent in hospital and believe me there were quite a few. On Christmas eve, the night nurses that were on duty would wait until we were asleep, or so they thought lol, then they would sneak in and put a big sack of toys at the bottom of our beds. Some of the toys were from our families, some from the hospital and charity organisations. Obviously, we didn't know that at the time, to us Santa had not forgotten us, and it was the magic of Christmas. All the nursing staff were dedicated to making it the best they could for us. They decorated the ward with streamers, balloons and we had a big Christmas tree, carol singers came, we had Santa Claus come with presents for us, and a special Christmas dinner with hats and crackers. We even had our own in-house pantomime, where the nurses and various hospital staff all took an acting part. It was presented in the hospital restaurant for all patients young and old. We got a real buzz if we recognised a nurse from our ward." Oh look" we'd say, jumping about with excitement "there's nurse Lake" etc. The fun was endless. I definitely got more in hospital than if I was at home. So, ask me where I would rather have been. I think you know the answer to that, no hesitation at all, HOME every time.

A few of the staff were outstanding and all these years later, I still remember them and exactly what they looked like. There was also the not so nice staff, horrible in fact, that I also still remember and what they looked like, thankfully these were few and far between. However, I will begin with the negatives then end on a positive note.

I am just going to give two negative examples, as these really were horrendous to me, and they certainly left their mark.

Two young female cadets, I would say in their late-teens, I don't know the organisation they represented or their names, just that they wore a pinkish uniform, they regularly visited us on the children's ward. This particular day they came to talk to me. I was in my bed when they came over, standing at either side, one of them started rummaging in the bottom of my locker while the other one kept me talking. I asked what she was doing and was told she was just tidying it up for me, it was days later I found out they had emptied my piggy bank, all the money my nana had put in for me they had stolen. I don't know why I didn't tell the nurses at the time; I waited until the Saturday to tell my mam. She went to see the sister but came back in tears because the sister just didn't believe it and obviously there was no proof. The thieving little toe rags, I wonder if they reflected on it in later life, such a despicable thing they did to a young child in hospital. Needless to say, we never saw them again.

This next person, I hated with a passion - she was the senior physio therapist in Saint Hilda's Hospital Hartlepool and the best word used to describe her was 'evil'. Obviously, I'm not going to name her even though I've never forgotten her name or her face, she had short blond tight curly hair and always wore those slip on Scholls on her feet, I remember that because I spent most of the time looking down at her feet 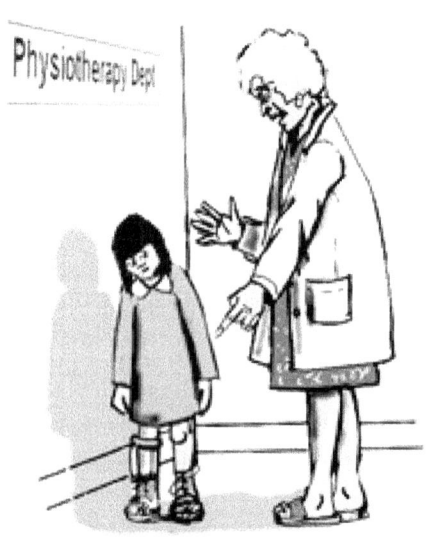 rather than her face. I will refer to her as Miss S. Once a week an ambulance would pick me from home or school for physiotherapy, and she would always be there waiting for me to arrive. To her, I was just a scruffy little kid from a council estate. I wore brown hospital surgical boots, and this is what she chose to focus on. As soon as I arrived, she would take me to one side and start shouting at me saying, "Look at the state of them boots, do you know how much they cost?" Then she would warn me that they had better be polished when I came back the next week. The main reason they were scratched and scraped was because I was forever falling over, and it was the way I had to drag myself back up. We didn't have enough money for food, never mind shoe polish. So, when I turned up with them in the same state the following week, and every week after that, it would be to the same telling off, then she would make me stand for an hour in the corner to wait for the ambulance to return, refusing me my Physiotherapy. Imagine the outcry if that happened today. It's funny I never ever told my mam about it, but I used to dread going, knowing what I had to face when I got there. This went on for a number of weeks, until the other members of staff began to notice, they would look over at me with a sad smile and a shake of their head, and so eventually she had to admit defeat, I guess this made her dislike me even more. The other thing I remember, she always made the old people cry, particularly the ladies, they were in terrible pain probably due to having severe arthritis. She would jerk their arms or legs up in a nasty manner saying, "Come on, you can get it higher than that." So cruel. One thing I am proud of, she never ever managed to make me cry, even though I felt like it sometimes. It's a pity we can't meet up with these people when we are adults. I think I would just tap her on the shoulder and say, "Hey remember me?" then proceed to punch her lights out. (Just joking). Anyway, in her case I would probably have to join a queue, lol.

Now for the lovely ones. I could go on and on with these, I've chosen a couple that were outstanding to me. There was nurse Lake, on ward 16 Sedgefield General. I remember her kindness when one time I had wet the bed. Normally when this happened to any of us, as it sometimes did, the nurses would only change the small draw sheet to get you through the night, then strip the bed fully the next morning. That's when all the other kids would know what you had done and would laugh and make fun of you. Nurse Lake said, "Right Pauline, we'll strip the bed now and no one need ever know." This was massive to me, and I've never forgotten it. A few years later when I was on the ladies ward, the same nurse Lake asked me if I could remember her. Apparently when I was a baby, she had taken me home with her for the day and had bought me a hat and coat with pom poms. How different things were then! It wouldn't be allowed now. Sadly, unlike the bed wetting incident, I was too young to remember but what a lovely, lovely lady.

Then there was Miss Russell, I think she was head of physiotherapy in Sedgefield General, now this lady I absolutely adored. She was small and chubby (if I'm allowed to say that) and always laughing. She used to regularly come and take me to her ward, not for physio but to play. The first thing she did was to take the callipers off my legs, and then she would put on knee pads for me so I could crawl and slide around on the polished floors. I absolutely loved it, and what a relief it was to be free from all that contraption. Then she would let me have a splash about in the hydro pool. Sometimes, unbeknown to anyone I would just leave the ward on my own and struggle down the corridor to see her. Her face would light up when she saw me and then she would try to tell me off for leaving the ward by myself, I always knew she didn't mean it. I loved her to bits, and I know she really cared about me; you just know these things, kids are very perceptive. All these years later, I still often think about my Miss Russell.

Now let me tell you about the Consultant Mr R Ellis. You will notice, I have no problem naming this amazing man. I was referred to him following the passing of Mr X. My first outpatient appointment with him was at St. Hilda's hospital in Hartlepool.

He took one look at me and said to his assistant, "Put her on that bed and get all that off her. I want to see what we can get rid of." Following his examination, he did away with the calliper on my left leg and the restrictive leather belt from around my waist that both callipers were attached to, it left me with just the one calliper on my right leg. This strengthens my belief that there was nothing wrong with my left leg, however it had become very weak, one, due to the unnecessary wearing of the said calliper for years, and two, due to the suspect procedures that he had carried out on that leg. Having only the one calliper was very strange and took some getting used to. That was when Mr Ellis arranged the weekly physiotherapy to help strengthen my left leg. It was to be my first introduction to the dreaded Miss S.

No longer was my mobility as robotic and restricted, however due to the above reasons, it was a real struggle to walk, my left leg being so weak, and so, as well as arranging the physiotherapy, Mr Ellis gave me a walking stick to help me adjust. I persevered, and although my left leg never fully recovered, it did eventually improve. Even though I would always rely on the calliper on my right leg, it was a sense of freedom of movement that I had never known. At this time, I was about 10 years old and so I had been under Mr. X's care for approx. nine years and during that time, he had performed numerous procedures that I still say were experimental and unnecessary. One such operation I remember involved me being in a full plaster cast, my left leg was completely encased, my right leg down to the knee, with the cast going all the way up to my neck, then I was literally placed on a wooden structure. Obviously I was flat on my back the whole time and I was like that for months. To what purpose, I have no idea. I have quite a number of ugly scars on both legs, and I have a twelve-inch-long scar running down my left hip, another across the top of my left leg, then numerous scars on my right side, including an eighteen inch one running the full length on the inside of my lower right leg. Each of the scars are a representation of a particular procedure and a lengthy hospital stay that not only robbed me of much of my childhood, but also the natural bond that is formed between a mother and her child. I also missed a large part of growing up with my brothers and sisters. Recently a friend of mine jokingly, asked my sister Marjy what I was like growing up. Her reply was, "I don't know, she was never there," I think that just about summed it up. However, despite all that, Marjy and me were not only sisters, but we also became great friends and soul mates, and we still are. Anyway, even though I managed without the calliper on my left leg, it would never fully recover, and as I said there has always been a weakness that has increased with advancing years, so much so that I am now a wheelchair user. If only I could have gotten my medical records from way back. For no other reason, but to confirm that my dad was right. Who knows, maybe a current orthopaedic consultant could shed some light on it.

Anyway, from then on Mr Ellis took me under his wing; he was a remarkably lovely man, and I trusted him completely. Obviously, there were no more procedures only regular check-up appointments. That is, until I was about fifteen years old, when he asked me if he could perform an operation to lengthen my right leg. If I agreed, although it would remain completely paralysed and I would always have to wear the calliper, I would no longer have to wear the built-up surgical boot. My right leg was two and a half inches shorter than my left. So it was a no brainer for me as I hated wearing the surgical boots and I agreed immediately.

We had to wait until he was sure I had stopped growing, then it was back to Sedgefield General Hospital for the operation. This time I was admitted to ward 5, the ladies ward. I think at a guess I was about sixteen or seventeen years old, and so, this was a whole new experience for me, having only ever been on the children's ward. But I'm happy to say, me being the youngest, everyone looked out for me, patients, and nurses alike. I remember one day; all the nurses were running around all excited. Apparently, members of the pop group Freddie and the Dreamers were in the hospital visiting one of their mothers. They were hijacked in the corridor by the nurses, bless them, and persuaded to come in and see me. They were absolutely lovely, but I was very shy, I just didn't know what to say to them. Maybe I should have just burst into song, singing their hit, You Were Made for Me. A blast from the past for those of you old enough to remember it, another memory I have kept.

Now to the dreaded operation to lengthen my leg. I can honestly say out of all of them I have had, that one was the worst ever, and I have never forgotten any part of it. I am not saying I was the first to ever get this operation, but it had to have been a relatively new procedure because after the operation other consultants would come with a team of trainee doctors to observe what had been done, obviously asking me first, did I mind? Anyway, back to the op. I remember I awoke from the anaesthetic crying, the pain I felt was like no other I had ever experienced, and I am definitely not a wimp. It was incredible what this operation to lengthen my leg involved, and it explained why I was in so much pain. During surgery, the shin bone was completely cut through, then the bone above and below the cut was drilled to accommodate four metal rods that were inserted, two above and two below the cut shin bone, they protruded from both sides of my leg and were attached to a full-length metal construction with two knobs on either side of it. I remember my mam cried when she saw the state of my leg.

Anyway, once everything had settled down after the operation, Mr Ellis came and told me they were going to start the actual lengthening of my leg. This was a shock to me as I thought it had already been done, talk about the worst was yet to come. A doctor would come to the ward twice a day, morning, and early evening to turn the knobs one full circle, this pulled the rods in an opposite direction separating the two halves of my shin bone, effectively lengthening my leg, the gap created with each turn of the knobs was miniscule and so, it took months to reach the two and half inches that was required. At the start of this knob turning, it was fine, a little but not too much pain, however as the time went on it got tighter and tighter, the rods were splitting the wounds that they were protruding from. This I could cope with, but the pain from separating and stretching the bone was unbearable, I was given constant pain relief morning and night, both tablet form and injection. Even with the pain relief, I couldn't sleep and used to cry silently through the night wishing I was home, it was so bad I begged the doctor to stop. Mr Ellis came to see me the following day and convinced me; we had got this far and so we had to carry on.

Once we had reached the desired length, it was months again waiting for the bone to grow and fill the gap. The progress of this was assessed by X Rays, each one showing how the bone was growing, only when the gap was completely filled was the contraption removed to be replaced with a full-length plaster cast. This was to allow the newly grown bone to strengthen. Finally, the day came when I was allowed out of bed. The whole procedure had taken a full year. I can clearly remember the day Sister McMann (another lovely lady) came to tell me I could get out of bed. I was so excited after being confined for all that time, she tried to hold back my enthusiasm telling me to take it slowly, but I was having none of it and was already sliding down the side of the bed. As soon as my left foot touched the floor (my good leg), pins and needles shot up my leg and the pain so bad, I actually collapsed; I cried out asking what was wrong. Sister McMann explained that it would take time and that it was to be expected due to my being in bed for so long. She sat me in an armchair by the bed and daily I would hold onto the arms of the chair and try to stand, I could only manage a minute or so at best, such was the pain. However I persevered because I was told as soon as I could walk with crutches, well hop really, as my right leg had not to touch the floor, I could go home, after which I would only be required to attend outpatients' for the removal of the cast when it was due. You don't need any more of an incentive than that. It took me about two weeks before I could stand and approximately four to fully weight bear and hop about on crutches. Even then it wasn't pain free, that took a whole lot longer, obviously after a year in bed there would also be muscle wastage. So, all in all, from start to finish, I had been on quite a journey, and definitely not one I would ever want to repeat. I hope I haven't bored you with that in depth description, but just the fact that I still remember every single detail, all this time later, tells you what? Well I think you know what I'm trying to say, so enough said, let's move on shall we? Lol.

When I look back, I can't help smiling because during the whole process I had point blank refused to look at or speak to Mr Ellis. He used to do his best to bring me round, telling me my hair looked nice, asking, had I done something different with it? Anything to try and get me to talk to him. After he had gone Sister McMann would shake her head saying, "Pauline, what you like? You're going to have to speak to him sometime." Then she would ruffle my hair and give me a hug. She not only knew what I had been through, she had been on the journey with me.

It was to be yet another Christmas spent in hospital and one of my presents was a guitar. Mr Ellis spotted it under my bed, and he asked me, did I want to learn to play it, I gave him a begrudging nod. The next thing I knew, he got his daughter to come and give me a couple of lessons. That's the kind of man he was, I still refused to speak to him though lol, then, when finally, it must have gotten the better of him, he asked me outright why I wouldn't speak to him.

I told him because he had tricked me into having the operation. He asked me, how had he tricked me? I said, "By not telling me how long it would take and the pain I would be in." He said, "And what if I had told you Pauline, what would you have done?" I said, "I wouldn't have bothered." He got hold of my hand in both of his, patted it, and said, "Exactly Pauline, and one day you will thank me for it," and of course, he was right. It was not the only amazing thing Mr Ellis did for me; I will explain later. That was the very last time I was admitted to hospital. All that could be done, had been, so apart from attending the Orthotics department when required for calliper repair or renewal, it was just a case of now getting on with my life.

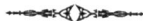

Growing up

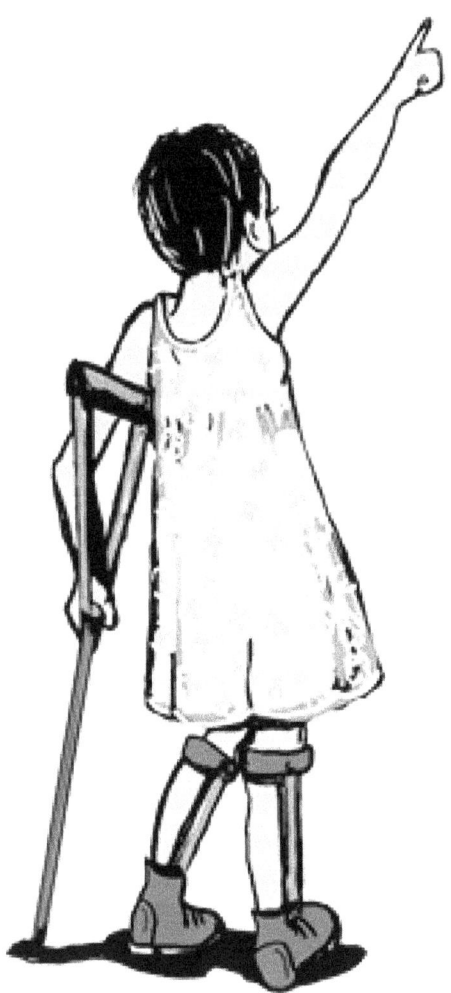

As I remember these were happy years, despite the poverty, deprivation and discrimination. I could even say, probably because of it.

So, yes growing up, where do I start? I will start with 25 Bowness Grove; it was the first home I remember, however it was not my mam and dad's first home. I remember dad telling us, if I've got this right, they started their married life living in a big house in Tweed Street, that they shared with other families. So, 25 Bowness Grove was their first real home together. It was a prefab in Hartlepool, the area was commonly known as Wagga. It was on the edge of an industrial estate. (Illustrated) not very picturesque I know, but hey you were just grateful in them days for a roof over your head and anyway, I can only ever remember being happy in all of our homes, that is, when I was at home and not in Hospital, because this was the time when I was a patient of Mr X. and subject to his numerous procedures I mentioned earlier.

I can just about remember living there, bearing in mind it was where we lived when I first got polio resulting in a lengthy eighteen-month hospital stay, that would have made me about four years old when I returned home. It was also the time when I struggled with the two full length callipers on my legs. It was so difficult to walk unaided, and I remember whenever I fell over, I couldn't get back up without help. We lived there until I was approximately ten years old, then we moved to 1 Scawfell Grove, those type of houses were, and still are referred to as the tin houses. The area was known as Belle Vue and it wasn't that far away from Wagga. Literally, it was just some waste ground that separated the two areas.

Something I nearly forgot to mention that was notoriously linked to the Wagga area, was the Wagga Dot. This was self-administered using a needle and Indian ink, so realistically it was a permanent tattoo. The dot was quite significant in size, and you would imprint it on various parts of your hands and face, one was usually on the top of the cheek, one on the v between your thumb and fore finger, or even a dot on the back of each finger. Thankfully, I was too young, so when I asked my sister Marjy who is nearly three years older than me, why she didn't have one she told me she wouldn't dream of permanently marking her face, or anywhere else for that matter, and that I better not be thinking about doing it either. She was my big sister, so needless to say, I didn't.

The funny thing was, my family moved house from Bowness Grove to Scawfell Grove, Belle Vue when I was once again in hospital, and they had been living there for quite a while by the time I was discharged. Well, I don't know about now but when I was a kid, council estates were pretty rough, I don't mean robbing and thieving rough, we weren't scallies. I mean survival rough, and I don't mean knives and stabbings, it was rarely heard of in them days, just good old fashioned fisticuffs. So anyway, if strange kids wandered into our domain, they would be questioned about their right to be there, then punched, and chased. Harsh, I know but that's just how it was.

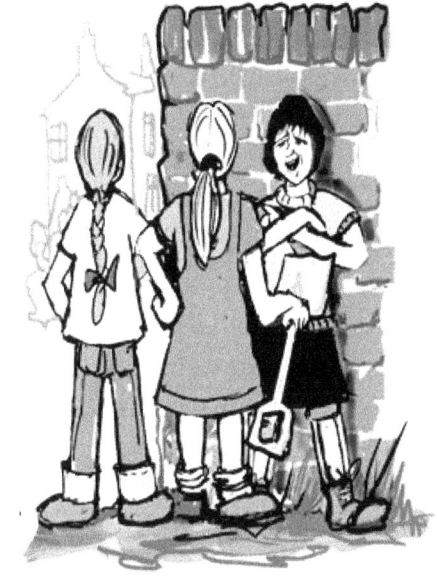

So, the day I went home from hospital, surprise, surprise, I was the strange kid who had no right to be there, or so they thought. I was stood on the corner of our grove minding my own business, leaning against the wall for support, when two lasses came over to me carrying a shovel. Why they were walking around with a shovel god only knows, anyway they pushed it in my stomach pinning me to the wall, asking me who I was and what I thought I was doing there. It went something like this: Them, "Wot you doing round ere?" Me, "I live ere." Them, "No yer don't." Me, "Yeh I do, I live in number one." Them, "No yer don't, the Roberts' live there." Me, "Yeh and I'm one of them so if you don't get that fucking shovel away from me, I'll wrap it round your fucking neck." They started laughing saying, "You'll be Pauline then?" I was home and accepted lol. So yes, surprisingly us kids swore then just like kids swear now, obviously not in front of any adults, risking a clip round the ear. And anyway, just because we were poor and swore a little, it didn't mean we weren't decent people. Everyone was in the same situation; the community spirit was second to none, and we all looked out for each other, a cup of sugar here, a couple of slices of bread there. I even remember when one of the neighbours got their electricity cut off, the neighbour opposite them, stretched an electric cable from the upstairs window over to their window just to help them out for a while. There was no messing around in them days, if you didn't pay your bills or your rent you were cut off or evicted, no matter how many kids you had. I also recall the times when callers came knocking, collecting debt money for something or other, my mam hiding and sending us to the door to say she wasn't in. We hated doing it knowing full well they didn't believe us. Just like the joke, "Well go and ask her, when will she be in?" Lol.

Our electricity was on a meter, I can't remember what coins were used but I do know some of the time if people had no money, they would try anything, like cutting up old floor canvas into rounds and using that, or metal washers, despite knowing they would be in trouble when the meter was emptied, and any money owed would have to be paid back. My dad used to tell us repeatedly, "The very first thing you pay, literally before anything, is the rent, it's the roof over your head and any way, if you can't afford to pay one week's rent what makes you think you can afford two the next week?" And so on, always wise words from my dad. So yes, we were poor and with seven mouths to feed, nine, counting mam and dad, food was sometimes scarce. The times I've seen my mam sitting crying because she had no money to feed us. I remember saying to her, "Don't cry mam we'll have jam n bread." No food banks in them days, although we did get free milk tokens. Occasionally through sheer desperation, she would send us round to my nana's (her mam). By this time I was down to wearing only the one calliper, so with my mobility being improved, I would sometimes have to go, my nana came across as a battle axe, but she really wasn't. We knew what to expect as soon as we went through the front door, it would be, "What do you want? If you've come for money, I've got none." Then I would say, "But nana me mam's got no money for our tea." "Well that's not my bloody fault is it? And it's no good standing there, I've got nowt." Whichever one of us it was, had strict instructions from mam, don't leave without any, so we would just stand there in the doorway for quite a while being ignored, before eventually giving up and turning round to leave, then she would shout us back, "Where do you think you going, here, and tell her it's the last bloody time." It was always the same old rigmarole, but we never left empty handed, bless her. Every Easter we all got an Easter egg and a bonny coloured boiled egg from her, and always a little something at Christmas. She did well really because we were not her only grand kids. We were, however, most definitely the poor relations.

My Granda was a funny man, always joking. I will never forget the day my nana was on at him to have a bath, he hated it, however he reluctantly agreed. It was so funny, when nana went to check on him, he had filled the bath with about six inches of water and was sat on the side fully clothed complete with cap, his trouser legs were rolled up with only his feet paddling in the water. Even my nana couldn't help laughing.

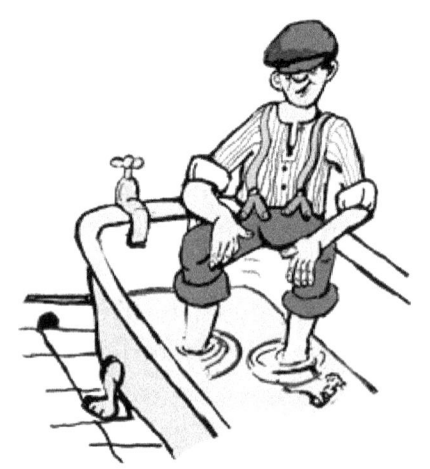

When I look back now at the life my mam had, all I can say is, that at the time we didn't really appreciate how hard it was for her looking after us all, I mean kids don't, do they? She self-sacrificed everything for us, and as if that wasn't enough, looking after us all, she also had a part time job cleaning. My dad was in and out of work, he was a contractor, and like most men in them days, he drank a lot, he wasn't exactly an alcoholic, but OMG he came home in some states. I think it was an escape from the sometimes hopeless situation the families found themselves in. It just wasn't fair on their wives. Where was their escape? I also remember the fights, it was very scary for us. It was always on a night when we were in bed. Me and my sister Marjy used to sit at the top of the stairs listening to them at each other's throats, then when it got so bad, on the verge of maybe becoming physical, one of us would go down crying, begging them to stop. It worked until the next time, again I think it was just the financial pressures they were under. My dad was very bad tempered, and at times he had no patience at all. He was very critical of us, his pet names for me and my sister Maureen, when he was in a bad mood was Ugg and Mug, not very flattering. I don't know if I was Ugg or Mug lol. I remember the nearest we ever got to a compliment from him, was when he regularly said, "Well, none of you are ugly." Wow don't hold back dad lol. I remember one day he was carrying me to Saint Hilda's Hospital for a check-up appointment. It was quite a distance away and probably due to him not having money for bus fare, he had to walk, and with the added burden of carrying me, he wasn't in a very good mood. The big button on his coat was digging in my leg and I suffered the whole of the journey in agony because I didn't dare tell him. I did tell him years later and I could tell he was very hurt. He said, "Bloody hell, I wasn't that bad was I?" "Yes," I said, "you were." I feel I have to say in my dad's defence, he wasn't always like that, and he definitely did not abuse us in anyway. I know he loved his kids and would have laid down his life for every one of us.

When he was in a good mood, there was no one better, he would sing to us, and as we stood on his boots, he would dance us around the room. But he was a no-nonsense kind of guy, and he would regularly say to us, "Don't come in here crying 'cos some one's hit you, or I'll bloody hit you," and so we never did. He was making sure we stood up for ourselves. Another thing he regularly said was, "Don't ever bring trouble to this door or you'll know about it." There was never a shortage of parental guidance or discipline, and in my opinion, we were all the better for it.

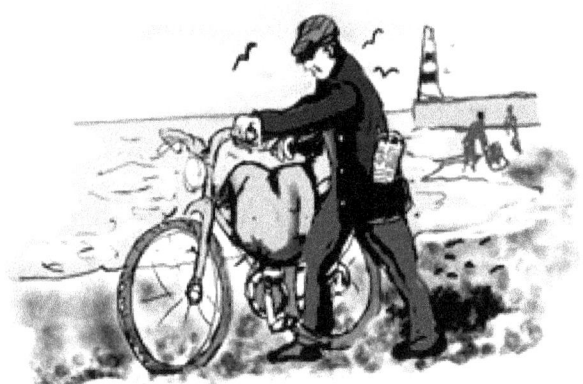

In our house the only form of heating in them days, was a coal fire in the front room, my dad had an old bike he would take down to the beach to collect sea coal, he would come back with three or four sacks at a time. He loaded them onto the bike and then manually pushed it all the way home. Looking back I don't know how he did it because not only were they extremely heavy, but it was also quite a distance from where we lived. So, as I said, good old dad, at times there was no one better. I remember us all sitting in front of the lovely roaring fire getting a warm, I also remember the hot missiles that used to spit out at you, landing on your bare legs, and us rubbing frantically to get them off lol. It must have been bits of shell or stones, a price we were happy to pay to keep warm. Another thing I remember about my dad, he was very intelligent, and he could compose a cracking letter, I can only describe his handwriting as beautiful. If any of the neighbours needed an official letter composing, he was the guy they came to.

I am sure you have heard it said a million times before, from people describing how cold it was in them days. It was when winters were winters, snow was a plenty, and as I said, the only form of heating was a coal fire in one room, even the inside of the windows would ice up. Well, let me tell you from one who knows, listening to it being told and living through it are definitely two different things. The windows were obviously single glazed, the frames were metal, and some of them were rusted, creaky and didn't close properly, so yes, they did ice up on the inside. We used to breathe on them then rub a circle so we could look out. After getting into bed, we would lie shivering for ages until it warmed up, then, on a morning, we didn't dare get out of bed it being so cold. We slept about four of us to a bed, top to tail, so snuggling up together helped us to keep warm. Sometimes in the middle of the night you would get a lovely warm sensation up your back, the warm very soon turning to cold, it meant someone had wet the bed, happy days lol. Oh yes, and the only toilet we had was outside, so we had a bucket that we could use through the night, obviously not all of us needed to lol.

Some mornings when we got up for school if the fire was not lit, usually because we had no coal, my mam would light the oven and leave the door open so we could sit round it and get warm. She would also have all our socks warming on the oven door. The things people take for granted now, like washing for instance, no automatic washing machines in them days, when my mam washed it literally took her all day, she had a single tub with an electric roller fixed on the back. Washing for seven kids and two adults, I remember the whole of the kitchen floor would be covered with piles of clothes and yes, it literally took her all day from start to finish. Then she had to get them dry. I'll never forget the day when she got her hand caught in the rollers, I remember her crying with the pain, her hand swelled up and turned black, but no trip to the hospital for her, she just struggled on to finish the washing. I can't ever remember my mam treating herself to anything except, in them days you could buy single sachets of Nescafe coffee. I used to see one of those sachets on top the mantel piece from time to time, so that was her one and only little treat.

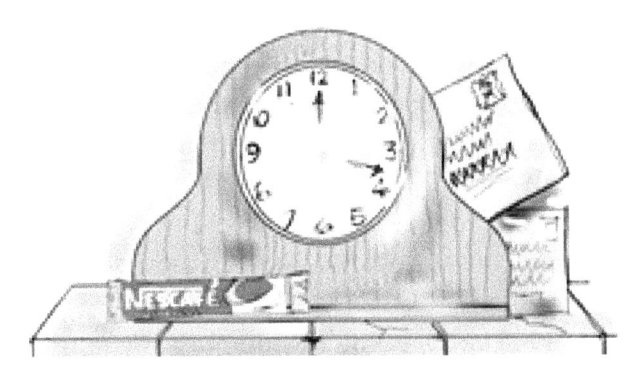

Also, permanently kept on the mantel piece was a wooden clock, the family hairbrush and a big comb, minus half its teeth. But, OMG that bloody hairbrush, it was the only one we had, and it serviced all nine of us lol. I remember if ever that bloody brush went missing off the mantel piece there was hell to pay from my dad. He would reach for the brush that wasn't there, then turn to us and say, "Where's the brush?" then when he got no response, he would shout, "Well bloody well look for it," then he would stand over us as we repeatedly opened and closed cupboards and drawers aimlessly revisiting the same places, and he would rant at us saying, "It must be the only bloody brush in Hartlepool with legs, well keep looking, go on, one foot in front of the other, it's called walking." The sarcasm was lost on us. Anyway, it always ended the same way, with us all in tears, and my mam screaming at him to bloody well get out if he was going out. Funny enough it always did turn up, so maybe dad was right, the only brush in Hartlepool with legs lol. Years later, my sister Marjy and me have had many a laugh over what we called the, 'Where's the brush saga'. It's good that we can look back on it in a humorous way. Happy days eh?

Then there was the nitty comb, it was made of steel, and it bloody well hurt. Mam used that on us once a week every Sunday after our bath, or whenever she saw us scratching our head. We still managed to get them from time to time, she used to crack them between her thumb nails then give us a clout for catching them in the first place, like it was our fault lol. Then it was out with the zulio (I think that's how you spell it), as I remember, it was a treatment that was used to eradicate them. At school we had what we called, the nitty nurse, we had to go to her and have, what us kids used to say, have our head looked. If she found any, we were sent home with a letter and couldn't return to school until we had treatment at the clinic and given the all clear. It was a constant battle, and all kids did get them at some point. I remember, my mam insisted on our hair being tied back for school to minimise the risk, so every morning we would line up with our bits of scraggy ribbon or a bit of bandage if no ribbon lol, for my mam to put it in a ponytail. OMG it was so tight it made your scalp hurt. Another thing that was rife in them days was impetigo, scabs/sores around the mouth, usually covered with bright purple ointment, not a pretty sight. I'm pleased to say I don't think any of us ever caught it. What I did suffer with every winter was chilblains on the back of my leg, I remember they were very itchy and sore.

Our clothes were usually hand me downs or clothes bought from the second-hand shops, nothing like charity shops of today, and we were always grateful for them. The only time I kicked off and refused to wear them, was when mam came in with some bottle green knickers lol, not because they were knickers but because they were bottle green. Everyone always wore navy blue ones and I remember a girl from school once turned up in green knickers and she was bullied and laughed at, so no green knickers for me. Mam was fine about it after I had explained. We did get new clothes once a year when my mam's provident clubs were due for renewal. Again, all spent on her kids, nothing new for herself. Through sheer desperation some of the neighbours on the estate sold their clubs for a lot less than they were worth just to get the ready cash, probably for food or to pay bills. A lot of the kids wore Wellies all the year round, and they sported the tell-tale, permanent black trademark Wellie rings round their legs to prove it. Wellies or shoes, it was the norm to have holes in them, we used to put cardboard inside to stop your socks poking through lol. Obviously not me, though I think I would have preferred them to the hospital boots I had to wear. At least you couldn't scratch, or scrape Wellies and it would probably have saved me from the wrath of the dreaded Miss S lol. In the winter our holey socks had another use, and that was on our hands as gloves when we played in the snow.

One thing I will always be grateful for growing up, was being treated just the same as my siblings by my parents. I was never wrapped in cotton wool because of my disability, no restrictions, exceptions, or privileges whatsoever and definitely none from my brothers or sisters. I can honestly say, I would not have wanted it any other way. The only exception to this was when I was first discharged from hospital, it was strange going home after each lengthy stay. I felt like a stranger in my own home, and I suppose that is exactly what I was, not having seen any of them for months and months at a time. My mam was lovely, she couldn't do enough for me, all smiles, loving having me back home, as was everyone else. It didn't feel natural though, everyone walking on eggshells around me. I am pleased to say it didn't last long, and so in no time at all, thankfully the above crept out, and normality crept in, and it was back to reality lol.

We had a lot more freedom then, than the kids of today. There were that many of us my mam was glad to get rid of us for the peace and quiet. Once, we were out, we only came back when we were hungry. Or as my mam would say, "Don't come back till teatime." The odd days that we didn't go out and play, we would sit indoors bickering, then, when we had pushed mam too far like fighting and arguing with each other, she would dash in usually from the kitchen and give us all a good clout saying, "I'm not bothered who started it, I'm bloody well finishing it, if it was raining, you'd all want to be out." Then she would return to the kitchen leaving us rubbing at the red hand marks she'd left, and needless to say, after that not a peep from any of us. I still think that is what is lacking today. It was a form of discipline, definitely not abuse and it did us no harm whatsoever. What it did do was teach us respect, and not to push the boundaries.

We never ever had a holiday, they were never heard of in them days, however, on very rare occasions my mam would pack up sandwiches and we would have a family day out, maybe to Crimdon Dene or Redcar, basically anywhere local you could get to by bus. I do remember one particular day out. It wasn't with my parents, it was with one of our neighbours, he was affectionately known locally as Pie Billy, probably because he was a very big man lol. Anyway, he had a horse and cart and because I was friends with his daughter I got to go with them to Appleby Fair. It was amazing, all the activities and attractions I had never seen before, the journey on the horse and cart was never ending such was the distance, but it was an adventure never to be forgotten.

Our meals were generally good wholesome food but cheap, like, for example, panackelty, homemade soup, mince and dumplings (with not much mince) Bubble and squeak, eggy bread, homemade rice pudding to name but a few, and whatever was put on the table, you bloody well ate it or did without. If we were really lucky, sometimes on a Sunday we would have a little cake each for afters, this was such a rare treat. They would all be different, sitting on a plate in the middle of the table, mam wouldn't let us have one until we finished our meal, so when she wasn't looking the quickest of us would grab the one, we wanted, lick the top of it then put it back saying, that's mine. No one else wanted it after that lol.

Usually for breakfast, my mam or dad would make us fat n bread, (as we called it). It was dripping, melted in the frying pan then the bread just dipped in it. it would be brought into the front room for us, on a big plate stacked high, it was lovely with tomato sauce, I can still remember the fat running down my chin. Another of our favourites was what dad called Pobs. It was bread broke up in a cup with hot milk poured over it, then sugar sprinkled on the top. We loved it but more importantly it filled us up, I guess that was the idea, we sometimes had that before bed. If we got hungry when out playing, we would sneak in the back door and help ourselves, (unbeknown to mam), to a slice of jam n bread, sugar n bread, sauce n bread, in fact literally anything you could slap on a slice of bread, then sneak back out eating it. The sneaking in and out was usually because it was in the early evening, so we were worried if mam heard us, she would keep us in.

We also found rhubarb growing wild that we would eat raw, we just pulled off a stick, dipped it in sugar and ate it, if you ate too much of it, you got a bad belly. I think the worst thing we ever did, I still cringe at the thought, was to scrape chuddy (chewing gum) off the ground with a lolly stick and eat it. When you think about it, it had been trod on, pissed on, and previously chewed by God knows who, but hey, we weren't bothered, and we lived to tell the tale. Funny enough, recently, I was watching GB News one morning when Nana Akua,(one of my favourite presenters) was speaking to one of her viewers who was politically fed up and said she was sick of eating the dirt that was being dished up by the government. I couldn't believe it when Nana said laughingly, "I've never eaten dirt, but I did use to scrape chewing gum off the ground as a kid." I couldn't stop laughing and nearly choked on my cuppa. She'll do for me.

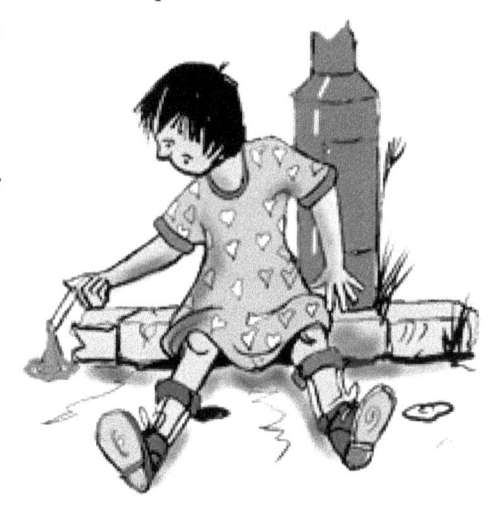

When I look back at some of the things, we did to entertain ourselves and how we had to improvise! For example, and I'm sure you will have heard of some of these things - making bogeys from pram wheels, planks of wood, nails and a length of rope. The front wheels of the bogey needed to be movable to steer, so we joined the two front pieces of wood together with a big nut and bolt. We didn't have a drill to make the hole, so we used a hot poker, we just stuck it in the fire till it was glowing red hot, then out into the garden to make the hole, we had to repeat the process numerous times before it actually made the hole, not exactly the health and safety of today, running through the house waving a red-hot poker about but hey, we knew no fear and it got the job done.

I have a tale to tell you about one of them bogeys we made. Me and a few of my friends, with my brother Kevin in tow, took one up a steep bank near to where we lived. I volunteered to ride it down the bank first; it had to have been one of the scariest things I had ever done. Usually, steering the bogey was done by your feet, but I couldn't do that, so I steered it using only the rope handle, obviously being roughly made by us, there was not the luxury of brakes. As I began my descent, I couldn't believe the speed it reached in such a very short time, it was almost immediate, the bogey was juddering and jumping all over the place, it was literally flying and I was terrified. How I managed to steer it to the bottom I will never know. Anyway miraculously I did, and because I did, my brother Kevin insisted on having a go, despite me telling him not to. You can guess the outcome, yep, Kevin didn't make it to the bottom.

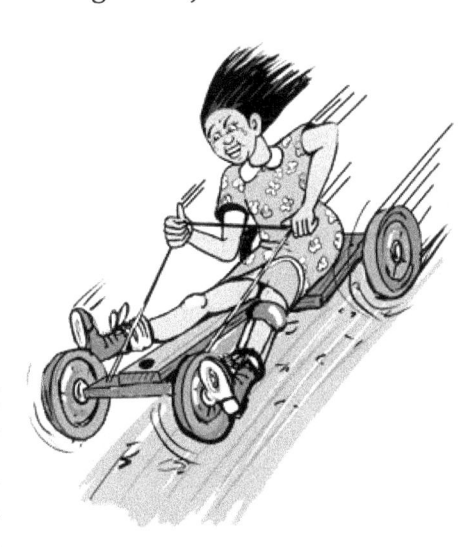

Halfway down the bank he lost control, the bogey flipped over, throwing him in the air, then him dropping to the ground with a thud. As well as being shocked, scraped and bruised, he had blood running down his face from a gash on his forehead. Luckily there was a hospital close by, it was Cameron's Maternity Hospital, so we headed there. A lovely nurse saw us and took us inside. She cleaned and dressed Kevin's wound and told us to take him straight home, which we did. Imagine that happening today. Hmmm, I think not, we would have been told it's not an accident and emergency hospital, then sent on our way. Anyway, Kevin still tells that story to this day. How I got down the bank and he didn't, a grudging respect for his sister maybe? I think not lol. Oh, and by the way, me being the oldest, I got the blame off my mam for allowing him to do it.

It was a similar story the first time I tried to ride a bike. My older sister had one, it was from one of the neighbours, he used to make them up from old scrap bikes and then sell them for a few bob. So, anyway, one day when she was out (cos she would've killed me) I wheeled it to the top of our grove and climbed on. Yes, as you can guess I just kept falling off, the problem was, my leg with the calliper on didn't bend so I couldn't turn the pedals, but I never gave up, and Hey Ho, a few hours later complete with my battle scars consisting of numerous cuts and bruises, but I'm pleased to say, no broken bones, I finally cracked it. I couldn't ride it the same way as everyone else did, something else I was about to get laughed at for, but I wasn't one bit bothered. Again, it was improvisation, I had to stand on the pedals, this meant I couldn't sit on the seat. I just used my right leg with the calliper on to press the pedal down then take it back up with my left leg so effectively the pedals only went halfway not a full circle, but it was enough to propel the bike. I was absolutely buzzing at my success until my sister Marjy came back to her battered bike. She took it off me and gave me a good clout lol. Such is life, but I was still buzzing. Guess what I wanted for Christmas?

For our entertainment we played group games like kick the tin, dodge ball, Itchy Bay, (you may know that as hopscotch), rounders, skips, we had a big, long rope that reached from one side of the grove to the other. It was so heavy it took two hands to turn, it was long enough for most of the kids to skip all at once. I always had to turn the rope because skipping, sadly I could not do, but I still enjoyed being a part of it. On rare occasions our mams would even join in, and we loved it. Another thing us girls did, we carried around in our pockets two small rubber balls, to play what we called 2-baller. It was just bouncing and catching them off a door or a wall, anything to keep us occupied at virtually no cost. We also used empty tins to walk on. We just put holes in the sides, threaded some string through to hold, then just stood on them and clunked about. I tried but just kept falling off, never mind, you can't win 'em all. Oh, and let's not forget the rope swings on the lamp posts.

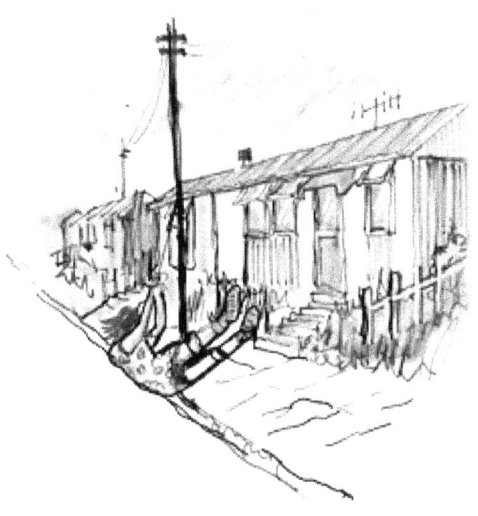

Occasionally, when my mam could afford it, we went to Seaton swimming baths. I loved swimming but I had a big problem, and that was getting from the changing rooms to the pool. All your clothes and belongings had to be put in lockers and that included my calliper. This meant I could not walk, and my left leg was not strong enough to hop. There were no disability facilities in them days, you were on your own, so literally, I would crawl on all fours, all the way from the changing room, through the foot bath to the actual pool. It seemed never ending and was oh! so embarrassing for a ten- or eleven-year-old, I hated doing it, but I loved swimming even more and so it was a price I had to pay. What a relief when I reached the pool, then, once in the water I was on par with everyone else. For as long as it lasted, I was no longer disabled, and I actually felt normal, well, let me tell you, it was a wonderful feeling, that is until I had to crawl back lol.

While I am with the Swimming theme, I have to tell you of an incident that happened when I was a few years older. I sometimes went swimming with my sister Marjy, she was about sixteen, making me around thirteen, she would piggyback me from the changing room to the pool, saving me the embarrassment of having to crawl, not that I would have at that age. Anyway, talk about embarrassment, what a laugh I had, this time it was at our Marj's expense. It was after we had been swimming a few lengths, we were sat on the side of the pool for a rest, dangling our feet in the water when a young lad swam over and he said to Marjy, "Hey missus, your cat's showing," she looked down and was mortified to see she was baring all, then she said, "Bugger off you cheeky little sod." I've never laughed so much, Marjy did see the funny side once she had got over the embarrassment. The trouble was, in them days our cossies (costumes) were made from seersucker, some were even knitted and so, when you got out of the pool they were filled with water and got distorted, they literally just hung off us, but eeh, it was just so funny lol. Anyway back to when we were little kids growing up. Sometimes we played naughty mischievous games like Nicky Nicky 9 doors. It was knocking on people's doors then running off without being seen or caught. Looking back I can see how annoying it would have been, it wasn't long before I found out just how annoying. Obviously, I couldn't run and so it would not be something I would ever do, but this one time the other kids I was with did it as we were passing. Without warning, they just knocked on two adjacent front doors and ran off leaving me standing there in a panic, so, some quick thinking required, I half climbed half fell over a low wall nearby and lay there hiding. Sure enough seconds later, two very angry men ran out of their front doors obviously used to it and fed up. I lay there shaking just feet away, listening to them ranting, "If I get my hands on the little bastards I'll wring their bloody necks." I was literally terrified because in them days it wasn't uncommon to get a well-deserved clip round the ear from an adult. I had to lie there until I was sure the coast was clear. When I eventually got back to my friends, I wasn't surprised to find them doubled up laughing, they just thought it was a huge joke, me, not so much, still feeling a little traumatised I wasn't one bit amused. I did find it funny later on though. Back then it wasn't just the adults we were wary of it was also the Bobby on the beat keeping order. Unlike today, we did respect our elders, definitely no back chat from us. There was always the fear that they would speak to our parents.

When I look back, it's a wonder we survived at all, especially me with my mobility problems, but I just ran ragged with the rest as best I could, as well as round the doors. Our playgrounds were the Tin Works, the Slag Banks, and Derelict Houses. The Tin Works were next to some railway lines, I remember seeing the open top trucks. I think they brought in surplus tin goods to be crushed. The reason I say that, once when we were there, we found one of the trucks full of cardboard boxes. Inside the boxes were sets of three beautiful biscuit tins, (unfortunately no biscuits), so we all helped ourselves to a box each. The tin works itself had high mountains of scrap tin waiting to be crushed, we would climb so far up them to see what we could find. It was sharp tin and so we would be covered in cuts and scrapes; and our clothes would get ripped to shreds. We didn't think we were doing anything wrong, to us it was just unwanted junk. One day we found all kinds of baking stuff, pudding tins, baking trays etc. that day every house in the grove got something, they were over the moon. We would just rummage around until we were spotted and chased by the workmen, usually shouting at us from the top of a crane. We would look about wondering where the voice was coming from, it usually went something like. "Fuck off you little bastards, if I have to come down there," etc. etc. These terms of endearment we were used to, just more of the same to us. It seemed everywhere we went, up to our usual mischief, it triggered the same old response. We would just scarper until the next time, me, as usual, lagging behind in my own fashion and pace.

I was ok in our own neighbourhood, accepted and just one of the gang, but it was a different story when we were out and about among strangers. As I said earlier, I have despised pity and sympathy all my life and I would get quite indignant if I heard it directed at me. From the adults it would be, "Aww look at that poor bairn" as if I couldn't hear them. On one occasion, when I was out with my friends, a lady ran up to me and stuck an ice cream in my hand. I knew she meant well but at the time I resented it. I remember my friends saying, "Wot she give ye that for?" I knew why but I wasn't going to say, as I said the lady meant well.

From other kids, obviously not from our estate, it would be any vile name they could think of, Spacca could easily have been my first name lol. Other names used were, cripple, mong, retard, freak etc. or they would mimic the way I walked. Funny enough I coped better with the kids' name calling and piss taking than I ever did with the adult sympathy, because at least I could react to the kids. It would begin with me saying the usual, "Come here and say that," I was never bothered about how old or big they were, girl or boy, it was all the same to me. Obviously, I couldn't catch them, so they would come over in a cocky manner, making the mistake of thinking because I was disabled, I was soft and incapable, but they very soon realised their mistake. The one thing I had in my favour, was extra upper body strength, effectively, my arms compensated for my legs so, on the ground I very rarely lost a fight, and if I did, it was pointless crying about it (remembering my dad's words) so

I never did, and anyway I could usually handle anything I was faced with, even losing a fight lol, mainly because I had always had to. That sense of survival, oh and not forgetting the pride thing as well. I have to say even though this name calling was upsetting at the time, I did survive it, and it made me stronger. I definitely don't agree with the namby pamby world we now live in where you can't say anything in case you offend, it is ridiculous. For me your childhood years growing up are when you grow the armour that sets you up to face the world of adulthood. Life is full of disappointments and sometimes heartbreak. It's no wonder millions of people suffer from anxiety and depression. It was never heard of in my day. Again, you just had to bloody well get on with it. Anyway, one particular fight I will never forget, it was over my brother George. Because of his learning disability he was constantly tormented by other kids, always to the point of tears. I was fiercely protective of him, and I still am, because I knew first-hand what it felt like, but unlike me, George didn't understand why, and he couldn't defend himself. Unlucky for this kid it was when I was older, about fourteen and he was roughly the same age. It was after I had learned to ride a bike and lucky for me, but not for him, I was on one that day. As I approached, I could see George, he was stood at our front gate crying and in a terrible state as this lad stood taunting him relentlessly, calling him all the horrible names I knew so well. I just saw red, and this was one kid I could chase and by God I was going to catch him.

When he looked round and saw me, being the coward

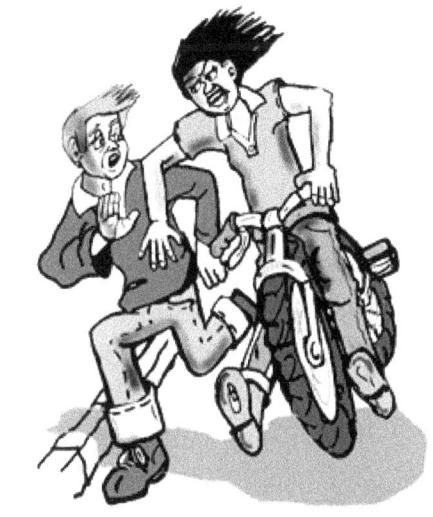

he was, he took off running down the road at full pelt. Lucky for me it was downhill, and so I managed to pick up enough speed to catch up to him, as I drew level. I was oh so angry, I threw caution to the wind and just dived off the bike grabbing him, crashing us both to the ground. I then proceeded to punch his face in telling him, "That's my brother, you bastard" All he kept saying was, "I'm sorry I'm sorry I'm sorry." I said, "You fucking will be if I ever see you round here again." I'm pleased to say, I don't think I ever did lol.

That incident was when we lived in Jesmond Gardens, so let's get back to my years living in Scawfell Grove, Belle Vue and the antics we got up to. I've already mentioned the tin works. Next I have a funny story relating to the slag banks. But hang on a sec, before I tell it, this fighting theme has triggered yet another memory and another scrap that occurred, not involving me, but surprise, surprise, my mam. She was arguing with the next-door neighbour, I can't remember why, probably a squabble over us kids. It was just verbal and would have remained so but for a certain nasty comment made by the neighbour. She said to my mam, "You're not normal you, if you were, you would've had normal kids." Well, talk about red rag to a bull, we knew no more. Mam jumped the fence and flattened her with one punch. Then she went back into our house and fainted on the floor. Mam was not a violent person and definitely not a fighter, but it was a case of, you can hurt me, but not my kids lol.

Anyway, so yes, the slag banks, as I remember they were two tiered. The low one, which was still quite high, we could just about manage to climb up. The kids used to crouch down on their feet, then using a piece of cardboard, they would slide down the bank. Obviously not me but I got a laugh just watching them. This day our Marjy's friend decided she would have a go. Unfortunately for her, halfway down the bank, her feet came from under her, and she slid the rest of the way down on her behind. When she got to the bottom her knickers were in shreds and her poor bum was all scraped and bleeding. I think inconsolable covers it; she ran home crying to her mam leaving us in stiches, luckily for her, she didn't need any, but it was quite a while before she could sit down, kids, eh?? We knew no fear lol.

Injuries such as these, and worse were quite a regular occurrence due to the environment we played in. For example, derelict houses were just like an adventure playground to us. We would go upstairs where most of the floorboards had been ripped up enabling us to shout down to our friends below, one slip and you could be joining them rather quickly. It was so dangerous, we could be messing around, when without any warning, half a building brick would come flying through the window, if the brick missed you, the glass didn't.

Unluckily for one lad, he got hit with a brick and was carted off to hospital in an ambulance with what looked like, quite a severe head injury. There certainly wasn't much left to demolish by the time we had finished so, if you look at it positively, maybe we were doing the community a service, eh?? Hmmm, maybe not lol.

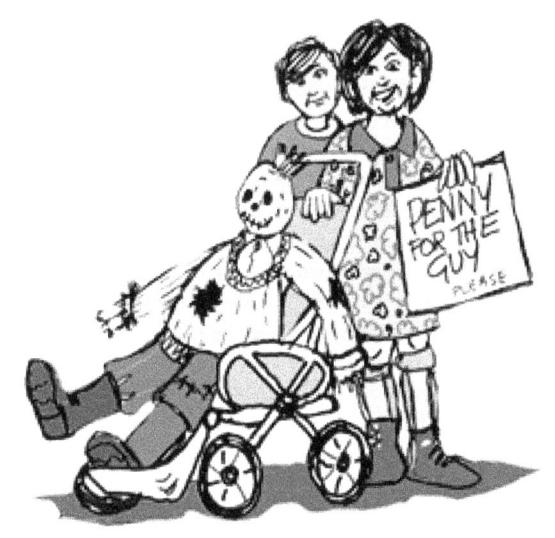

We never missed an opportunity to try and make some pocket money. Christmas time, it would be carol singing, wintertime we would go snow shovelling, clearing paths and drives at private houses. Bonfire night it was penny for the guy, we made the guy ourselves using an old pair of trousers and a jumper stuffed with scrunched up old newspapers, the head was made of anything we could find. We usually started collecting about a week before. The money we made, we used to buy fireworks to set off around a big bonfire we had on the common. We had spent weeks prior collecting unwanted items and newspapers from neighbours to build the bonfire. We would take the guy to our usual spot, our spot being the Belle Vue Social Club. I remember one particular time when we were there, it was on a Saturday night, and as we stood just outside of the entrance, we heard this lovely music, so we all dashed over and looked through the window, eager to see where it was coming from. There on the stage we saw this beautiful lady in a long blue sparkly dress, her arms were raised up as she sang out. We were just stood there glued to the spot, staring at her in awe, mesmerised, when one of our neighbours, who was about to go into the club, came over to see what we were looking at, then he turned to me and said, "Well you know who that is, don't you Pauline,"? "No," I said, "I don't." "Well, it's your auntie Mim. Your dad's sister." I was shocked as I had never set eyes on her before. But seizing the moment to show off, with my head held high I nudged my friends saying proudly, "Hey that's my Auntie Mim," lol. Of course, they didn't believe me. When I got home, I mentioned it to my dad, and yes it was true, she was my dad's sister, Miriam (Mim for short) and yes, she was a professional singer, part of a group of entertainers called the Mellow Maniacs. (Illustrated) It wasn't until years later that I saw her again, and sadly it was at my dad's funeral. I'm pleased to say, we had a lovely chat. Oh, and yes, I did happen to mention to her the night I saw her on the stage, she thought it was hilarious. I don't know why they lost touch. Sadly families do for one reason or another, and our family was and is no different, but I do believe, and I am pleased to say, that they did reconnect during the last few years of my dad's life.

So that was pretty much it for Bowness Grove and Scawfell Grove. We moved to Jesmond Gardens when I was about thirteen, and yes, this time I moved with them. My mam and my sister Marjy went to view the house, and they came back buzzing with enthusiasm. Mam, couldn't believe we had been offered the house, one, it had four bedrooms and two, it was in a lovely area, directly opposite Grey Fields, a recreational/pavilion sports park. Funny enough, I wasn't as enthusiastic, yes it was lovely, but I would miss my friends, and with us being new to the area, it would be back to the name calling etc. however it didn't last long, and I settled in relatively ok. The day we moved in, we discovered a massive problem, the house had an infestation of Blacklock beetles. Apparently, all the houses had them. They came out at night when the house was in darkness, then as soon as the lights were switched on, they scattered away in all directions, it was so scary. If we did need to enter after dark, we would sneak our hand round the door, switch the light on, quickly close the door then wait a few minutes until they had dispersed lol. One day, my brother George, (if you remember, I explained to you his learning disability), well he was sat in the armchair, and happened to see one on his knee, he immediately stood up, flicked it off and from that day forward he never ever sat down in the living room again, preferring to stand behind my dad's chair to watch the television, sometimes, actually falling asleep on his feet. Thankfully my dad did eventually get rid of them by drilling holes in the floorboards and dropping down smoke bombs. However, it made no difference to George, as no amount of persuasion could get him to sit down ever again in that room.

I did say earlier that Jesmond Gardens was directly opposite Grey Fields recreational park. Well, every Saturday and Sunday football and rugby matches were played there. I remember on one particular Sunday, I was sitting in our front bedroom brushing my hair when suddenly, crash bang wallop, a rugby ball came crashing through the window, it bounced off my head showering me with glass lol. A few minutes later a very embarrassed guy came to our door apologising profusely to my dad assuring him he would pay for the damage. It didn't stop him from asking for the ball back though lol. Dad was fine about it and I wasn't hurt, I actually found it very funny.

Now then, I did say earlier that accidents and injuries were a common occurrence in our daily lives growing up, well I think this next incident could top the lot. I was travelling home with a few friends following a day out at Seaton Beach. We used to go regularly, armed with our jam sarnies and a bottle of council pop (tap water) to see us through the day, then we would get the bus home, but because we never had enough money we would only pay so far, and just stay on the bus. Generally the drivers knew what we were doing and would just turn a blind eye. Not this time though, as soon as we got on his bus, this particular driver was a grumpy old sod, so, no surprise when we got to the stop we had paid for, he basically threw us off. I'm not saying we didn't do wrong but looking back, he had to have been kind of heartless to throw a disabled kid off his bus, again, not looking for sympathy, just making a point. Anyway, needless to say we got off rather sharpish and had to walk the rest of the way home.

We hadn't got far, when there, in the middle of the pavement lay a bright yellow object, it was metal, round, and it had two straps, one on either side, I picked it up, wrapped it round my wrist and said laughingly to my friends, "Look it's like a big watch." Then I took it off, put it in my jeans pocket and forgot about it. That is until later that day, I was in our back garden with my brother Kevin when I remembered it in my pocket. I got a hold of it shook it, and something inside it rattled. Curious as to what it was, I put it on the ground, and I spotted the chopping axe that we used to chop fire wood, I decided to use that to try and open it up. I hit it twice, the first time it bounced off the second time there was this almighty bang, it had exploded in my face, I was reeling, dazed and in shock, not knowing what had happened to me. I will never forget the look of horror on my brother Kevin's face as he stared at me. I couldn't feel my face at all, it was numb, then when I touched it, my hand was covered in blood. At that point, my mam came running out, took one look at me and started shouting at me in panic, "What the bloody hell have you done?" She said as she pressed the tea towel that she had in her hand firmly onto my face to stem the bleeding. One of the many neighbours that had run outdoors to see what had happened, had called 999 and I was rushed to hospital with the blue light flashing. You would never believe it, but the object we had found, turned out to be a railway detonator. The explosion had ripped open the left side of my face. At the hospital, they stitched and dressed the wound, then I was allowed home. I was sat in the chair watching TV trying to eat a bag of crisps on the good side of my mouth, when my sister Marjy came running in sobbing, staring at my face, asking if I was alright. I just said to her, "What you crying for, I'm ok." Kevin, who hadn't seen me since the explosion, had met her off the bus, and had told her I had blown half my face off with a bomb lol. It did actually make the front page of our local newspaper. The headlines were *'Girl hits Railway Detonator with Chopping Axe'* lol. A couple of days later I went out with my friends to Seaton when a man, having noticed the dressing on my face,

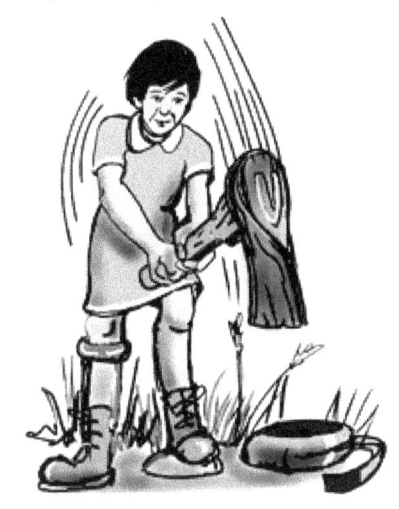

actually stopped me to ask if I was that girl, fame at last lol. Anyway all joking apart it left me with a horrible large scar on my left cheek, that crinkled up when I smiled, it was awful, and I was devastated.

Do you remember me saying earlier that there was another amazing thing Mr R Ellis did for me? Well, it was this - when I went for a check-up appointment with him, not surprisingly, the first thing he noticed was the scar on my face, he couldn't believe what I had done. He told me his friend was a plastic surgeon, and he asked me if I would like him to have a word. Well, that is exactly what he did, and not too long after, I had the surgery, the result was a remarkable transformation. I have so much to thank that man for. Oh, and obviously, not forgetting his friend the plastic surgeon, I think his name was Mr Choudry, who had very kindly and expertly obliged his request and I remain eternally grateful.

That was going to be the end of this section titled, Growing Up, but after confiding in a friend and getting advice as to whether I should or should not include a very personal and traumatic thing that happened to me, we decided that yes, I should include it. I have kept it a secret all these years, and have never spoken of it ever, until now. So here goes. It happened when we lived in Scawfell Grove, so I would have been aged around ten or eleven. It was early evening, and I was outside our front gate playing with a set of pram wheels, basically, it was the bottom half of an old pram, and it helped me to get around. Well, I was just standing there when I was approached by a man. He asked me if there were any back streets nearby cos, he needed a wee, (his words). I did say we had an outside toilet if he wanted to use that, he obviously said no, so I pointed over to where the back street was. He asked me if I would show him. As you can guess being an innocent kid, I did as he asked. When we got there, he grabbed me and dragged me behind a bin or something, then he exposed himself, he grabbed hold of my hand telling me to touch it, I was terrified, I tried to pull my hand away, crying and saying repeatedly, "I don't want to." The ordeal went on for quite a while, him making me touch it saying things like, "Come on, it won't bite you." Until lucky for me, a lady came out of her back yard and saw us, it startled him, and he had to let go of me. I wasted no time at all. Grabbing my pram wheels I dashed home as best I could. I was so traumatised as I sheepishly crept into our house and sat on the couch shaking. My mam took one look at me and said, "What's wrong with you, what have you been up to?" "Nothing mam," I said. Why do kids in these situations think that they are to blame? I certainly did and to this day I never ever told my mam or dad what had happened to me. I dread to think what the outcome would have been, had that lady not appeared when she did. I can't help thinking, what a lucky escape I had that day.

So, on that scary reminiscent note, I really will end this section called growing up and quickly move onto my school years.

My School Years

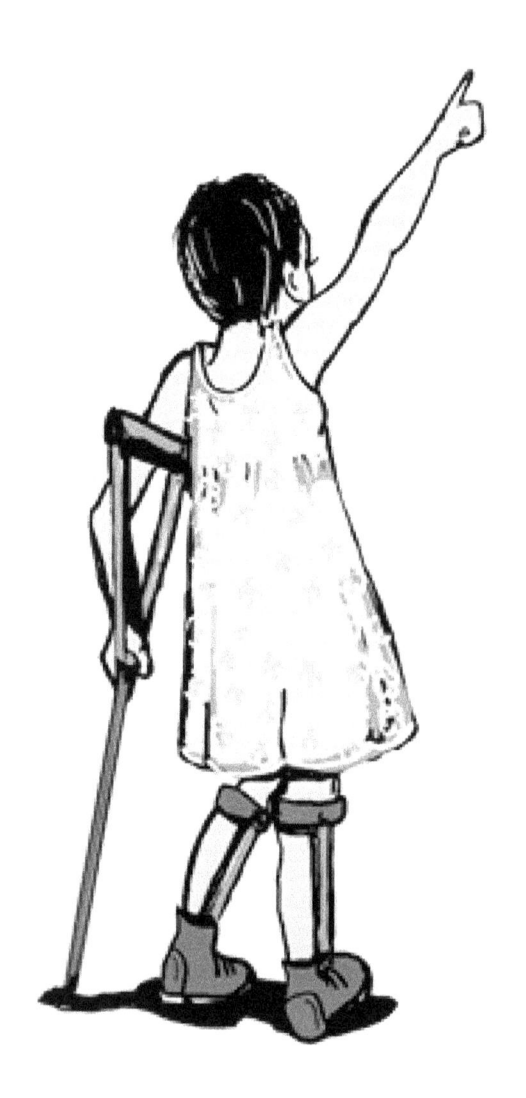

Yes, very happy years I spent at the Thornhill Open Air special needs school. However, sadly my education was disrupted due to my frequent hospital stays.

I can honestly say, I loved school. Unlike present day, when it would be classed as discrimination, back then parents of kids with disabilities had no choice, they were automatically sent to a special needs school, and I was no different. In my case though, it was probably for the best when you consider the amount of schooling I missed, due to my lengthy hospital stays, I would have been so far behind, mainstream school would almost certainly have been a struggle for me. So, the school I attended was Thornhill Open Air school. You remained in the same school throughout your learning years, just changing classrooms and teachers as you progressed, until leaving at the age of sixteen.

I did a little research and apparently, the school was built back in 1935 specifically for delicate and disabled kids. All the classrooms were individual buildings with floor to ceiling glass windows on three sides, making them light and airy. The school was situated in the countryside, hence the name, the Open-Air school. In fact, weather permitting, some lessons were taken outdoors. It was also a requirement for infants and juniors to have an afternoon nap, once a senior it was no longer a requirement. So, straight after dinner we would all toddle off to what was called the bed shed, all the beds were set out in rows, I do believe some years previously, even the beds were used out in the open air. Anyway they were just like camp beds, low to the ground, made of tubular steel and covered in canvas. We each had our own blanket and pillow; they were kept in a cubby hole with our name on it. I do remember we had a strict lady assistant that used to supervise us throughout the rest period. She would make us stand by our bed with our arms down by our sides, then proceed to wrap the blanket around us as tight as she could so we couldn't move, we gritted our teeth in dreaded anticipation as she picked us up and plonked us down none too gently onto the bed, sometimes missing the pillow and hitting our head on the top bar. I don't think it was intentional, and not hard enough to cause harm but not a very pleasant experience just the same. Then, that was us for the next hour or so. I think I spent most of it trying to wriggle out of what I can only liken to a bloody strait jacket, and that was most definitely intentional lol.

I don't think many of us actually went to sleep, however we just had to lie there, with not a peep from any of us. After a time, which seemed to go on forever, it was everyone up, beds stacked against the wall, blankets and pillows rolled up and shoved back in our cubby hole, then off to the classroom for our afternoon lessons. As education goes, it wasn't exactly mainstream, no exams at the end, although some of us did sit the eleven plus, which, not surprisingly, I failed. So, no qualifications, but I certainly have no complaints, the teachers were dedicated to doing the very best they could for us, which at times, can't have been easy due to the various support needs that some of their individual pupils required. One good thing, we didn't have to wear a school uniform. As I said, I loved school, but there were a few downsides, one of them I remember, you were made to feel uncomfortable if you were having free school dinners, and on occasion the teachers would ask us, not IF, your dad was working, but WHERE, is your dad working? hoping to catch us out if we were claiming them fraudulently. My answer was always the same, "he's not working miss" strict instructions from my mam, lol. Sometimes he was, sometimes he wasn't, but working or not it was still very hard for my mam, trying to make ends meet, so it was always the same answer. Regarding free dinners, I'll never forget one particular day, we were all in the dinner hall, when the head stood up and actually said, "All those who pay for their dinners can go and get seconds." Imagine the outcry if that happened today. I'm pleased to say, it only ever happened the once, I think in hindsight he must have realised it was a mistake. I just remember sitting there, squirming in my seat feeling very uncomfortable. As I said, it only ever happened the once, he was actually a lovely man, and we all really liked him. As for the school dinners, it wasn't that I wanted seconds, I actually hated the dinners, it was just the being made to feel worthless really, watching the other kids come back to the table with their second helping, smirking at us.

In my very early school years, I was a little scrawny kid, and was often referred to as little Pauline. The least thing would make me sick, for example, lumps in the mash, fat or gristle in the mince, skin or lumps in the custard, I just couldn't eat it without retching. Sometimes the same strict assistant from the bed shed would be on dinner duty, and she would keep me back after everyone had gone, to try and make me eat it, but it was a waste of her time and effort, because even though I tried, I just couldn't. As an alternative form of nourishment, I remember being given a spoonful of malteline every day, sticky sweet brown stuff that I actually did like.

Every year we had a sports day, there wasn't much I could excel at. However, no one could catch me and my friend Janet in the Wheelbarrow race lol, obviously, I was the wheelbarrow, and it was great fun.

We also had PE, I can remember the big heavy medicine balls, the vaulting horse, the exercise mats etc.

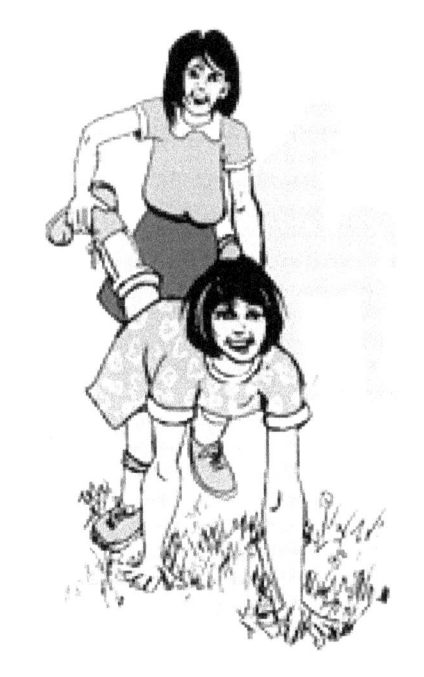

I loved PE. Obviously, there was a limit to what I could do, but I was game for anything. Somersaults, and standing on my head, posed no problem at all. We had a monkey rope hanging from the ceiling and the kids would climb up it, gripping the rope with their knees, I'm proud to say I could climb to the top using only my hands lol.

We used to go for swimming lessons one afternoon a week. This was not at the public baths, it was a smaller pool at one of the Schools, I can't remember which one, but what I can remember, thankfully, such was the setup, the only crawl I had to do was the swimming stroke lol. I remember there was a requirement that the girls had to wear a swimming cap. Well, I didn't have one and my mam couldn't afford to get me one. So, when I explained to our headmistress of the time, why I couldn't go, she bought one for me and let me pay it back at threepence a week. Her name was Miss Smart, and she was lovely. One of the highlights of school for me was, when we went to Carlton Camp for a week, holidays were unheard of, and so, what an amazing experience that was. I can remember the dormitories and the bunk beds we slept in, that in itself was an adventure. It was endless fun. On a night, we had a right carry on, pillow fights, fun fights etc. Until the teachers came, and in the nicest possible way, not wanting to spoil our fun, they resumed order and settled us down for the night. We had a full week of indoor and outdoor activities. Oh, and not forgetting the last night, it was incredible, we had a farewell party, and we were all asked to get up individually and do a turn. I'm proud to say, I sang the song, My Favourite Things, from the film, The Sound of Music. The teachers knew I loved to sing, and so I was picked to do a solo in the village church, but because I didn't have the confidence to do it on my own, they asked another girl to sing with me. We sang the Lord is my Shepherd, it was so special, and such a memorable occasion for both of us. There isn't much more I can say about my school years, we did the usual lessons, beginning with the basics, reading, writing and arithmetic, these, obviously being the most important, particularly reading, because it opens so many doors and gives you the ability to research, resulting in additional self-learning. I have been an avid reader all my life, and that, in itself has been a learning curve for me. It has also helped me to fill in some of the gaps I had in my education, due to my frequent hospital stays.

So yes, just to round up this section, I did love school, and there were some benefits to attending a special needs school at that time, one of them being, the fact that each and every one of us having a disability or a health issue, meant inclusion and not being made to feel like an outcast. As for the leaving without any qualifications, I'm pleased to say, it did not hold me back at all. My training and qualifications came later. Sadly, the teachers that taught me, almost certainly are not here now. If they were, it would have been a privilege to pass on a sincere and heart felt thank you from me to each and every one of them.

Before I leave this section, does anyone remember the thunderstorm of all thunderstorms that hit us in July 1968? I was fifteen and at school, I have never forgotten it. At around lunch time, suddenly everything went pitch black. Fork lightning lit up the sky, then came giant hail stones, and torrential rain, OMG it was so scary, we all thought it was the end of the world, even the teachers were very worried. The headline in the Evening Gazette read, Midnight at Midday.

Working

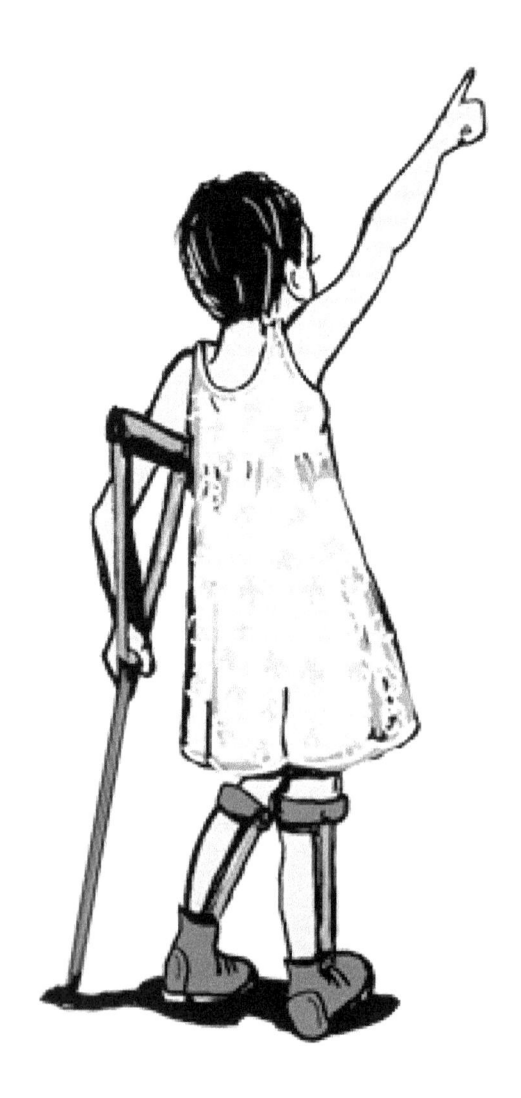

So yes, my world of work, this section in particular sums up everything. The values and influences instilled in me by my dad, the love and the sacrifices I witnessed and benefitted from my mam, and the hard lessons of life growing up. In my opinion, all these attributes set me up to face the world of adulthood and identified the person I became.

In our house, it was never an option not to work or not to pay lodge money. I can still remember the pep talk from my dad, he said, "We've brought you up, fed and clothed you as best we could, now it's your turn to give a bit back." And he was right so yes, definitely no complaints from us. I can't remember exactly how old I was when I started work, it all depends on when I had the operation to lengthen my leg. Seventeen or eighteen, certainly no older than that. We had a Careers Officer in them days and I remember her taking me to my first interview. It was at John Colliers, a textile factory dealing in menswear, suits, trousers, jackets etc. As I recall, the interview didn't go that well. I was told I wouldn't get anywhere until I lost the chip off my shoulder lol. So never having heard that phrase before, I asked her, "What's a chip, oh and on which shoulder?" I think she found it amusing and must have seen some potential in me because she gave me a little smile, and yes, surprisingly she gave me the job. In my defence, as I said it was just that I didn't know what the term chip on your shoulder meant, and I was always on the defensive. Anyway, unfortunately I was set to fail, because being left-handed I couldn't be a machinist and as that was the only sitting down job in the place, unbelievably, and wait for it, I was given the job as a runner, you couldn't make it up, could you? Lol. I had to keep the machinists stocked with work, it meant I was on my feet all day humping and carrying bundles from section to section, constantly at everyone's beck and call. I gave it my best shot but unfortunately, I only lasted a week because at the end of each day, my leg had swelled up so badly and

I was in agony, so yes, I had to give it up. From there, I got a job at GEC Telecommunications working as a Relay Adjuster. This was a sitting down job, perfect really, but I found it boring, so after about 6 months I heard Buxted Chicken factory were recruiting. I told my mam and she said, "You won't last five minutes in there," well it was a bit longer than that, 14 years to be exact.

When I look back, it is with some regret and a feeling of hypocrisy really, that I, being the animal lover I was, could work in such a place. I can't really explain it or excuse it except to say, that when you are young you take a different approach to life. Although I did have some guilt, I told myself it was a food source, and it was just a job. I wasn't a vegetarian then although I am now and have been for the past twenty-five years. Also, the part of the factory I worked in, they came to us pretty much oven ready, so I didn't actually see them alive. Still not an excuse I know and something I have had to live with. I think conscience and regret comes on reflection in later life, it certainly has with me.

Anyway, for my sins I did work there, the conditions were not good, and even though the pay was way better than anywhere else, they still struggled to recruit and retain staff, which was lucky for me really as I don't think I would have been considered had this not been the case. So yes I got the job, however it was not without some concern. For example, the department I worked in was ankle deep in water, and that was a problem for me. I couldn't wear the wellies that were provided, and so there I was working away in my own shoes, when the section supervisor came over to me, he put his arm around my shoulder and said, "aww look Hun, your feet are soaking wet." I said "Oh, don't worry I'm not bothered, its ok." "Aww no Hun, we can't have this," and he walked away. Oh well, I thought, that's the end of another job, so I waited to be summoned to the Personnel Officer. However, after about an hour had passed, the same supervisor came back to me. He had taken the trouble to go out and buy me a pair of waterproof overshoes, a lovely act of kindness from this man, enabled me to keep my job. The girls I worked with were the salt of the earth, and the camaraderie was second to none. However, it was extremely hard work, and as I said, not in the best of conditions and so, definitely not a job for the faint hearted. What I remember most was the laughs, and believe you me, they were a-plenty. Here are a few examples I think, worth a mention. On our section there was an ice pit, and in it was a machine that churned out ice. Well, this day me and my friend Cath climbed in for a bit of a skive, when a few minutes later we heard the chargehand calling our names looking for us. As Cath quickly climbed out, he shouted, "Where the hell have you been, and where's bloody Pauline?" At that precise moment, I lost my footing, slipped down the bank of ice, straight through the hatch and landed on the conveyor belt, "Here I am" I said, as it carried me along. It was meant to be a telling off, but he couldn't do anything for laughing.

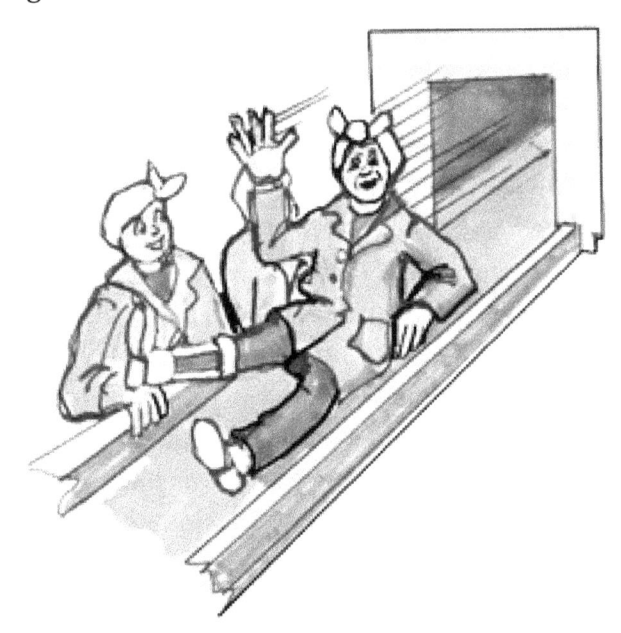

Another funny moment involved a lovely guy called Brian; we all loved him he was a laugh a minute, he reminded me, for those of you who remember, the comedian Eric Morcombe, of the Morcombe and Wise double act, right down to the black glasses. Well, this day I was working away, minding my own business, when he came over to me and said innocently, "Pauline, can I ask you a question?" I replied, "Of course you can Brian." Then, with not a hint of a smile he said to me, "What size tits are you?" for just a second or two, I was taken aback, gobsmacked, then we locked eyes and just fell about laughing, "Bugger off Brian," I said, "none of your bloody business," and that was the end of that. The funny thing was, sometimes the lasses were worse than the lads, all in good fun though, and no one took offence to it.

I mentioned earlier about the water on the floor, well not only the water it was also greasy making it quite slippery. Well, you know what I'm going to say, yes, I was on my backside more than I was on my feet. It was such a regular occurrence, I didn't realise how much this was seen by everyone as the norm for me, until the day I was walking along with my friend Cath. We were deep in conversation when I suddenly slipped, and down I went. Cath stopped in her tracks, looked down at me as we both just carried on with the conversation, I got up and we walked on as though nothing had happened. Looking back, I find this so funny. The thing is, over the years, whenever I did fall, I very rarely hurt myself, I do believe that, as it was such a regular occurrence growing up, I had actually learned how to fall, minimising the risk of hurt or injury.

Another thing we did every day was to sing, it was usually me that started it off. We were a section of young girls, and we used to raise the roof, the older women loved it as much as we did, they regularly said, "Come on Pauline, get the singing going."

There was a memorable event that took place sometime in the 70's and that was a wage robbery. In them days we were paid cash in a pay packet, multiply that by approximately 500 employees and it would certainly equate to a substantial amount of money. It was an inside job, and as I remember they had a lookout guy who had to whistle the tune, Yellow River, to warn them that someone was approaching lol. However, it did not succeed, I believe all the money was recovered and the guys involved did go to prison. I remember a post card was sent to the factory from one of the guys saying, having a nice time, wish you were here. We all had a bloody good laugh at that. I have tried to research the robbery but could not find any reference to it. It's like it never happened, but I know it definitely did. It's not something you would forget, especially when your hard, earned wages have been nicked lol.

So, all in all it was happy eventful years I spent there. However, there was a downside for me working at Buxted that I hadn't taken into consideration, and that was the distance I had to travel. The factory was situated at the other side of town, and so it involved me getting two buses. I got the first bus to the town centre where I caught the next one to the factory, then it was quite a distance I had to walk from the bus stop, and because it took me a lot longer than anyone else, I had to start my journey ridiculously earlier to compensate and to ensure I wasn't late. It was bad enough in the summer months but OMG, the winters were horrendous for me, because of the snow and ice, but I never ever considered it an option not to go. There was one good thing that came from me travelling so early.

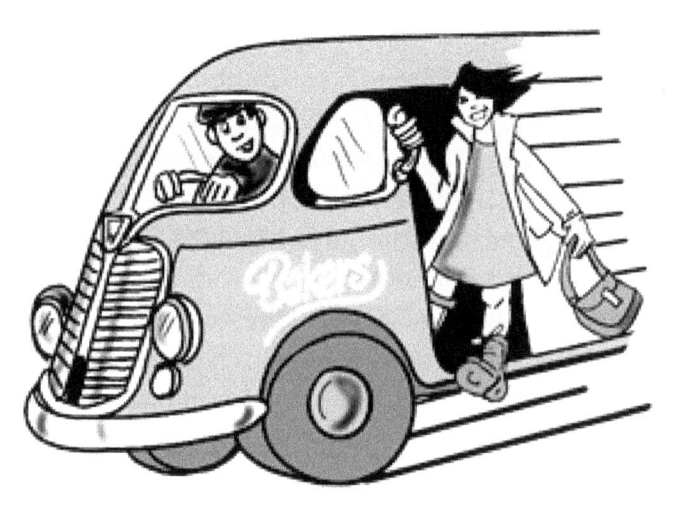

A bakery van was making a delivery around the same time, and I have never ever forgotten the kindness of the amazing, lovely man that drove that van. The first morning he saw me, he pulled up alongside and said, "Hop on love and I'll run you round." He did that every time he saw me. I just can't stress enough what that act of kindness meant to me, but unfortunately, he didn't deliver every morning, and the times he didn't pick me up, I remember being really stressed, particularly as I said, during the winter months. At times I was actually reduced to tears, it was so cold, and such a struggle for me, it was bad enough when I fell, but it was even worse trying to get back up in the snow and ice. However, everything has a positive, and so, in one way it was a good thing, because through the stress and tears, I made a vow to myself that one day I was going to have a bloody car and that became my only focus, well, more of an obsession really, I could think of nothing else. Well, eventually I achieved my goal, but even that was not to be straightforward. I couldn't get driving lessons anywhere because the driving schools just didn't have automatic cars, it would have been impossible for me to drive a manual having the use of only one leg, so, it was the cart before the horse for me. I had to buy the car first, before I could drive, and then learn in that. To get the car, I worked every hour I could, starting at 7.30am, then after my own shift ended, I stayed back and worked overtime with the evening shift finishing at 9pm, this was most weekdays. I even got a barmaid's job working weekends. This was thanks to my friend Sarah, she worked at the Seaton Social Club, and told me they were looking for someone to start, so she took me along for an interview. The Stewardess took one look at me, shook her head and said, "I don't think so pet, you won't manage it." Her husband jumped straight in and said, "Hang on a minute, we've got Betty there, hobbling about like a drunken duck, so give her a chance." The Betty (not her real name) he was referring to was an older lady. She had a bit of a limp, his words were not exactly politically correct, but hey ho, we didn't worry too much about that in them days, the main thing was, I got the job, and yes it was a hell of a struggle, but I was determined, I had a beer crate behind the bar that I could sit on now and again for a rest and that got me through. It was all work and no play with very little sleep, and as a result, I actually suffered with nervous tension for a while, but yes, I was determined to have that car, and I could think of nothing else. I worked and worked, saved and saved, until finally, the big day came. As I said, way back then, there were no small automatic cars so, my first ever car was a Wolseley 1800, and what a beautiful car it was. I viewed it, I loved it, and I bought it, at a cost of around £600. That was a lot of money in them days, and I had saved every penny. It was dark green with a lovely chrome trim. Obviously, it wasn't a new one, but I was oh so proud of that car, I couldn't believe I had actually achieved what I had set out do, and oh what a difference it was going to make to my life. Funny enough, I never did get any driving lessons, I went out in the car a few times with qualified drivers, my brother-in-law being one and various friends. I had also bought a book on driving, that I had read cover to cover repeatedly. In less than two weeks I was driving around town a fully confident driver, and I'm proud to say I passed my driving test first time.

OMG, I can't even begin to describe fully the amazing difference that car made to my life. It was sheer joy, no more getting two buses to work at ridiculous times in the morning and, more importantly no more having to walk round that dreaded road in all weathers. Needless to say, as a priority I have had a car ever since. I have to say though in them days it was sometimes a financial struggle to maintain a car on the wages I earned, and so, at this point, I will mention years later, the introduction of a benefit from the government called Mobility allowance. My dad made the application for me and after attending a medical, I was successful. It later became DLA and is now known as PIP. All my cars since, have been via the amazing Motability lease scheme and I am eternally grateful for this, it is the only benefit allowance I have ever claimed. Having a reliable car has definitely helped me to continue working all these years, and me now being a wheelchair user, over seventy years of age and still working, I make no apology for it.

Actually, while we are on the DLA theme I may as well tell you of an upsetting incident that happened to me a few years ago. I had gone to Scarborough with friends for a few days. I parked my car in the Grand hotel car park. Then on the day of departure, I went back to my car on my mobility scooter to offload my luggage. Unfortunately, the car in the next bay had parked so close, I couldn't open the door fully. The only way I could access was to gently, and I say again gently, rest my car door against his. Suddenly I heard a voice behind me say, "Excuse me, what do you think you're doing? That happens to be my car that you are damaging," then he went on to say, "oh but you won't be too bothered will you, probably not worked a day in your life getting everything on a plate." OMG I couldn't believe what I was hearing. "Actually" I said, "you couldn't be more wrong, I've worked all my life, and I still do work and anyway, who the hell gives you the right to make those assumptions just because I'm disabled." I think the final word was 'Off'. Despite the fact that he then quickly scuttled away with a red face and a flea in his ear, I did find the altercation very upsetting, it got me thinking. Did everyone look at me as a benefit scrounger? Oh, and by the way neither car door was damaged at all. So, following that unpleasant little snippet, let's get back in time to the job at Buxted. As I said I worked there roughly for fourteen years, until one day at the end of our shift we were called into the canteen for a meeting, where without any prior warning we were informed that the factory was closing down. It actually closed in 1981. Over 500 people lost their jobs. Everyone was in shock some were even reduced to tears. My worry was, I had just got a bank loan to buy, you've guessed it, a car. Not to be beaten, me and my friend Sarah found out there was a Buxted factory in Aberdeen Scotland. We wasted no time on preliminaries, just packed a case each, threw them in my car and that was that no forward planning, it was Scotland here we come lol.

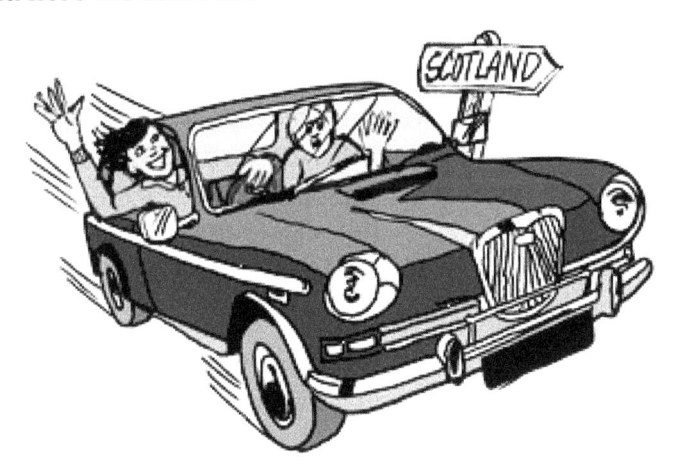

As we drove into Aberdeen, we came across a caravan site. I said to Sarah, maybe there is one to rent, we saw a young girl standing at her door watching us and I asked her the question, she said yes, the one next door to her was empty, then she informed us that the friend she was sharing with had left and she couldn't afford the bills, so she came and shared with us. It was a better outcome than we could ever have hoped for, it was so far so good. The next thing was the job, we wasted no time, just drove straight to the factory to enquire if there were any vacancies, and due to our years of experience, they took us on. We were buzzing. In just one day we had made the journey, had somewhere to stay and more importantly, we had found a job. It was happy times we spent there, the Scottish people were very friendly, and we were made welcome. It was a four-day working week, Monday to Thursday, this enabled us to go home most weekends.

I stayed for about six months, after which I began to get homesick and so I returned home. That was the only time I was ever unemployed, and I hated it. In desperation, I visited the jobcentre every day. On one such visit, I was informed that a company called Remploy were looking to employ a person to work on the electronic section, the said person would need to have soldering experience, and so I agreed to go on a three-week training course at Billingham college. I was willing to try anything to gain employment again. By this time I had been unemployed for about two months. At the end of the course, I had to assemble a circuit board against the clock using my newly acquired skills and take it with me to the interview as a sample of my work. I'm happy to say, I got the job, and it was to last me the next 25 years.

Remploy was a government subsidised organisation consisting of around 90 plus factories throughout the UK employing people with disabilities. The Hartlepool factory did subcontract work for various companies like Black and Decker, and Nissan. The work ranged from simple packing jobs to semi-skilled and skilled work such as electronics, cable harness and loom assembly, paint spraying and metal work. It may have been government funded, but it functioned in exactly the same way as any other factory in manufacturing, the same rules, regulations and expectations applied. All the jobs were time based and so we worked to a bonus system. There were also the usual grievances from the shop floor and the management that needed resolving, and as I had taken on the job of Union Rep. this was largely down to me. Even though it was at times very stressful, it was a responsibility that I relished. I like to think I earned the respect of, not only my members but also the management, this was due to the fact that I was not a militant, I just strove for fair play on both sides. I will give you an example of this, I was called into the office with one of my members, he was about to get a warning for his appalling absence record, Remploy offered a very generous sick pay allowance scheme, and it was open to constant abuse. Anyway as we sat in the office, the manager tore him off a strip, I offered no defence as it was well deserved. When we came out of the office, he said to me, "Bloody hell Pauline, I thought you were on my side," to which I replied, "Listen, I am on no one's side, I'm on the side of right, and right's right and wrong's wrong no matter who is doing it, and you are taking the piss, so shape up or you are going to lose your job." Equally, if management were being unreasonable, I would go all out on behalf of my members, here is an example of this. It was a Monday morning, and I was working away on my own when the production manager came up to me smiling as he asked, did I have a nice weekend? I replied that yes, I did thank you, but being as I didn't think it was the reason for him being there, what was on his mind? What followed, was too long and drawn out, so I'll give you the short version. He thought we were taking too long over our breaks and wanted to enforce a bell to bell working. Basically, don't leave your job till the first bell goes, then be back at your bench prior to the second bell, and all this to be achieved in just 10minutes. Seb Coe would have struggled with it, never mind disabled people. "You have to be joking," I said, but no, I could see that he wasn't. "Ok then let's give it a go," I said, "we'll start with me shall we? Tomorrow I will do as you ask, at break times I won't leave the bench till the first bell goes, then I will return to my bench prior to the second bell." His face lit up until I informed him of my second intention, that currently I worked at the high 90 minute hour work performance, but, as a consequence of his request, I would drop my work output to a 30, minute hour with immediate effect and in addition to that, I would advise my members to do the same. I then asked him, what did he think he had achieved, other than a drastic drop in production. It got very heated resulting in me winning the argument, and him storming off, saying, "I thought I would have had your support with this, Pauline," to which I replied, "Well clearly, you haven't." Just at that, a head popped up from the other side of the high-backed work bench, he was a member and unbeknown to me, had heard every word. He said to me, and I quote, "Fucking hell Pauline, I know now why I pay my union dues," then we proceeded to have a bloody good laugh about it. Needless to say, bell to bell working was never mentioned again. So yes, all I wanted was fair play in the workplace, and I think I achieved it, gaining respect from both sides.

We had a number of employees that were profoundly deaf, and one of the things that bothered me was, whenever they had a grievance that they needed to discuss with me, it was always with an interpreter present. I felt this denied them the same level of privacy afforded to everyone else, and so I decided to learn BSL (British Sign Language). Although my achievements were nowhere near to that of an interpreter, I'm pleased to say, it was adequate enough to enable me to converse with them on a one-to-one basis.

After about fifteen years, the day eventually came when I decided that I had had enough of the constant grievances, confrontations, petty squabbles and yes, mediation, so I did resign the position. My members surprised me by contacting a radio station to express their gratitude and to thank me on air. It was an unforgettable honour for me, and for them to let me know that my services were appreciated made it all the more worthwhile. Also, I was surprised and a little embarrassed to see that an article was published in the local paper. Not long after my resignation as a Union Rep. Remploy introduced a new and exciting initiative to the business called Interwork. It was an opportunity that was open to anyone who had a disability or health issue and were looking to gain employment. Not in the Remploy factories, but in outside industry.

> **Hard work**
>
> AN EMPLOYEE is celebrating after receiving an award to mark over 15 years of hard work as part of a worldwide disabled day.
>
> Pauline Roberts received a Making A Difference at Work award for 17 years' service at Remploy's Hartlepool manufacturing unit.
>
> The shop floor union representative was presented with the award at a ceremony to celebrate the United Nations International Day of Disabled.
>
> Remploy manager Dorothy Hancock said: "The award was presented to Pauline for all her hard work at Remploy over the years.
>
> "She has just been promoted and received the award for her role as shop floor union representative for the workers.
>
> "The award is presented to those people who have made a difference by improving their own or other people's working lives."

Pauline Cares A Lot!

A CARING business woman has been recognised for her superb support of her employees. Pauline Roberts, of Hartlepool, had been nominated by her colleagues for a Making a Difference at work award. It is the second year running that Pauline has been nominated by Remploy. She was commended for improving conditions on the shop floor and has so far this year helped seven disabled employees into outside full time work. Remploy's Manager Michael Connor said: "Pauline goes from strength to strength and is dedicated to improving the life of her disabled colleagues. She is a valuable asset to the company.

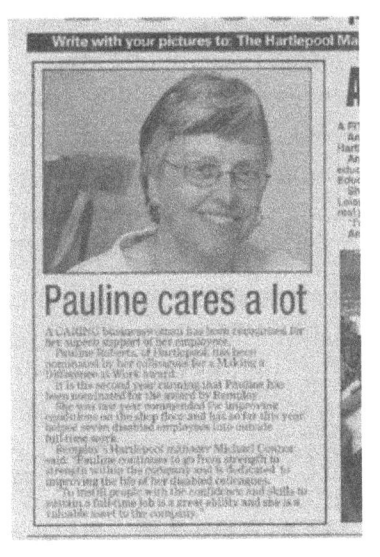

The applicants were referred to us from the jobcentre, they were then invited to attend an interview, to establish their goals and aspirations, but in the main to determine how serious they were about wanting a job as we did get time wasters just playing the game, even then. Remploy support included, training, job search facilities, job trials, interview techniques, basically just about anything that was needed to support the clients into sustainable employment. To the prospective employers, the support we offered could be practical, financial or both. When a vacancy came up within Remploy for an Employment Advisor, to work with, and deliver all the above support. I was tempted, but it was quite a promotional jump for me, from the shop floor, and I wasn't sure, so I asked my manager at the time, did she think I was capable of doing the job, her reply was, "Standing on your head Pauline," and so I applied. I knew I was up against it; in fact, I learned afterwards that I was a rank outsider that had been granted an interview just as a formality. I put my heart and soul into preparing for that interview, then, finally the big day came. I was so nervous, that as soon as the introductions were over, I literally just froze. I sat with my head down staring at the floor, barely answering the questions that were being asked of me, that is, until I looked up and saw the expression of disbelief on the faces of the two interviewers, it said to me, what the hell have we got here? That was the wake-up call I needed, I took a moment, gave my head a shake and said to myself, Pauline, you fucking idiot this is a once in a lifetime opportunity, so at least give it your best shot. After which amazingly, I did get the job. One of the two people that interviewed me was a lady called Lesley, and she became my manager. The feedback she gave me from the interview was, that they gave me no chance at all until suddenly I opened up like a flower (her words) and immediately after, Lesley wanted me on her team, I'm pleased to say I didn't let her down.

It is probably the most rewarding thing I have ever done. My past knowledge and experience as a union Rep proved to be invaluable, particularly when dealing with companies, helping me to overcome discrimination and negativity towards disability. Also, the fact that I myself had a disability meant I could relate to the people I was supporting and gain their trust. It proved to be a very successful programme. I don't know the exact number of people that not only gained employment, but with the ongoing support given, a large majority of them retained their jobs, and I do know it made a significant difference. I worked as an employment advisor for ten years after which, at the age of fifty-seven or fifty-eight I took early retirement. At last, some me time, I was free to do all the things I wanted to do. It was great to begin with, then gradually it was a steady decline for me. Most days I just sat watching daytime TV, and if I was not going out anywhere, I wouldn't even bother getting dressed. It was not too long after that, I started to feel down and depressed, it creeps up on you, a feeling of no self-worth or purpose, then thankfully, the day came when I thought to myself, this is no good, I need to do something about it. That something was for me to try and get another job. It's funny how things turn out, I went to a Mobility shop to buy myself a scooter when on impulse I asked the guy serving me, if the owner was available, to which he replied, "Yes, I'm the owner." His name was Ian, "Oh right," I said, "then it's you I need to speak to, are there any jobs going?" He shook his head and said sorry not at the moment. I informed him of my past work experiences, that I was in no hurry, and I asked him, would he just keep me in mind? To be honest, I didn't give it much hope, and at that moment in time I would have gladly worked for nothing. A week later, I had a message on my landline from him, informing me that my scooter was ready for me to collect, oh and would I like to have a chat about the job. That was then, and this is now, fourteen years later at the age of seventy-one, I still do work for this very caring, family-owned business, and I love it.

So, there we are, that was my life growing up, a life complete with all of its ups and downs, a life that I am really proud of. I say again, I am especially proud of my mam and dad, for the sacrifices they made, bringing us up against the odds. It also sums up the fifty plus years so far, of my working life. It has made me the person I am today.

So yes, the person I am today? Well, I am single, I decided very early on that married life was not for me and despite having three proposals of marriage, during my lifetime, I have remained single. I also never wanted children, as they say, none to make you laugh, none to make you cry. I think partly, it was because I witnessed first-hand the sacrifices made by my parents, and the hard life they had that made them old before their time, so it was not for me. I have never regretted either decision. Well, if I'm being honest that's a little bit of a lie, I did actually regret declining the first proposal, we were young and he went on to marry someone else. I actually kept his wedding photo from the Hartlepool Mail, it was splashed with a tear or two. But you can't dwell on these things just as you can't turn the clock back. I am my own person, I'm strong willed, I'm enjoying the life I have chosen for myself, and I don't answer to anyone. So yes, in the main all in all, no regrets.

You will remember I mentioned earlier I love to sing, well, I am proud to say, I am a member of the Hartlepool Community Choir. I love our weekly practice sessions. George Colley is our music director, we all love George, his expert tuition, his dedication and determination, all applied in his endeavour to make us the best we can be, even his reprimands and telling offs are tinged with humour collectively making it such an enjoyable experience. The singing is so uplifting, and everyone is so friendly and welcoming. The highlight for me is the three or four concerts we perform each year, it is such a privilege to be a part of it.

However, there is another event that by far surpasses all else and that is the yearly remembrance Sunday that we are invited to attend. I am actually reduced to tears whilst singing as I recognise the ultimate sacrifice that was made by many. A debt that can never ever be repaid.

The other thing I mentioned was my love of animals, well my kids have always been the furry, four-legged kind lol. I have always had dogs. My present baby is called Dolly, and she is adorable. They are non-judgemental, their loyalty is unwavering, and they just love you unconditionally. The downside is the fact that their life expectancy is way shorter than ours meaning inevitable heartbreak will come when they go, in response to this I gain comfort in the belief that it is not about them dying, rather than the life they have enjoyed, and my knowing I always did my very best for them.

Before I end this section, I will leave you with a final quote from my dad. He said to me, "Pauline, if you go through life never deliberately hurting anyone, doing a good turn whenever you can, you won't go far wrong." Well, that is what I have always tried to do.

So, I did ask that you read the book in its entirety and now having done so, hopefully you have come to the same conclusion that I have, that there is no comparison of how things were then, to how things are today. The generous welfare state we now live in has virtually eradicated the level of poverty that we experienced. However it is open to abuse, the evidence being the unacceptable high numbers of people not in work, claiming benefits and as such, enjoying a free quality of life that is far superior to the life of poverty and hardship that I, and most of the people I grew up with experienced. As a consequence of this, sadly the pride has gone, what we have now in society is a feeling of expectation, entitlement, and privilege, even if we have made no contribution to deserve it.

So, I say again, make your own life choices, be responsible for them and stand by them.

Stop Whinging and Just Get on With It.

Present Day

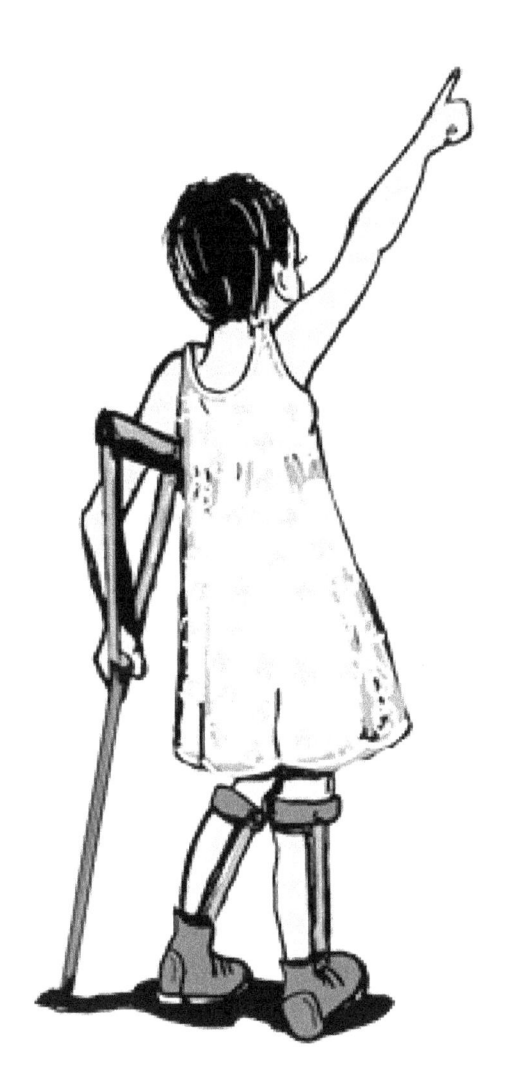

Yes, I feel there is plenty to say regarding where we are today, I'm afraid to say it is mostly criticism, so here goes.

So yes, present day. This is now and what do I think of our present situation? The answer to that is NOT MUCH, despite the poverty the deprivation and the discrimination I experienced that barely exists today, I would happily return to them days in a heartbeat. I will now explain why I feel that way and to share with you how I see things today. I accept not everyone will agree with my views, but here goes.

I will start with, OMG where has my country gone? The country I was born and raised, the country I was so proud of now broken, and devastatingly I see no way back. What or who do I blame? That's easy, weak and at times pathetic governments past and present running the country into a steady decline. The last fourteen years of a, so called Conservative party, that has lost its way, and the Labour party before that. I actually voted for the Conservative party, despite coming from a devout Labour household. I always vote for the party that I feel is the best suited to run the country at that particular time. I expect heavy criticism when I say the best prime minister for me in my lifetime was the iron lady, Margaret Thatcher. Now there was a leader with backbone, capable of making a decision no matter how unpopular it was and sticking to it because she believed in it. I accept she was not always right, but come on, who is? Importantly she was patriotic with an unwavering love for her country. She was a prominent global figure that was needed and never more so than now. I say again this is just my opinion, however given the fact that she won three consecutive General elections, I guess I'm not alone.

We are in desperate need of a leader with similar qualities, someone who is not afraid to fight for, and maintain our rights as a country. To recognise what is happening, and to do something about it, we need action, not empty words. We are losing our values, our traditions, our culture even our freedom of speech. We are becoming second class citizens in our country.

So now for the things I feel, we really should -

Whinge about, as loud and for as long as we can.

Out of control immigration is the main thing that is on every one's mind, and no, I am not a racist It is just about the unsustainable numbers. I say again it is out of control resulting in over population exhausting all of our essential services. Why on earth has this ludicrous situation been allowed to happen, or more importantly, when is it going to end? The short answer to that is, it won't. Can I just say, France is laughing at us, and we are actually paying them for the privilege? It's madness but then again if the tables were turned and they were leaving this country by the thousands, would we really want to stop them?

Even our national flag is frowned upon. Can I propose we have a National Flag Flying Day, Union Jacks as far as the eye can see, and no, again, this isn't racism, it's called patriotism?

Crime is out of control, innocent people are being murdered in the most despicable of ways, so many that it is no longer the shocking news it used to be. Shoplifting and burglaries are not worth investigating. I feel we are on the verge of a lawless society. We no longer feel safe on our streets. I could go on and on, but I think you get where I'm coming from, and I would be very surprised if you didn't agree with me.

Another problem we have, that can't be blamed on immigration is the amount of people claiming benefits. Since the Covid pandemic it has been announced that the amount of people claiming has reached an unsustainable level. I say again, there are disabled people that genuinely can't work, and they should most definitely continue to receive their well-deserved ongoing support, no question. However, unfortunately there are malingerers out there that are cleverly playing the system. Oh no, I hear you say, and to that I say, come on be honest, we all know someone, friends or family that have been doing it for years, absolutely nothing wrong with them other than an aversion to work. Unfortunately, they are jeopardising the future wellbeing of genuine disabled people, present and future, as they are the ones that will undoubtedly be caught up in any future clamp down.

Then we have the NHS, it's a drain on the public purse, and definitely not value for money. In my opinion, this is largely due to mis- management. It's a service that is not fit for purpose, a steady decline over the years, beginning with far too many highly paid managers, I have relatives and friends working for the NHS, and even the customers that come into the shop where I work, all say the same thing. Why can't we have a government with the courage to seriously investigate and modernise an essential organisation that we quite simply value and cannot do without?

One of my biggest criticisms of today's NHS, aside from the long waiting lists and the impossible task of getting a dentist, is the lack of care and compassion particularly towards the people of advancing years. I have even heard of them, whilst being hospitalised referred to as bed blockers, how sad and disrespectful is that? The decline is even apparent in our GP Surgeries. Gone is the caring friendly family doctor, sadly to be replaced with cool indifference, clinical diagnosis, with hardly a look never mind a kindly smile, all delivered alongside an imaginary clock that is tick ticking away, making you aware that your allotted ten minutes are about to be up. Oh and don't even think about mentioning a secondary condition, you will be told this requires another appointment, and this, at a time when you are feeling your most vulnerable.

Let me explain my particular reason for losing faith in the NHS. Where do I start? When I compare the nursing staff that I knew and experienced, to today's equivalent, there is no comparison at all. In my day it was a vocation, they cared for their patients' every need, nothing was beneath them, always putting them first. So yes, why have I lost faith? Well I will tell you. It concerns a lifelong friend and soul mate of mine. Her name was Rosemary Carter, and personally I will never ever forgive some of the nursing staff on ward four of the James Cook Hospital in Middlesbrough, for the way they treated her. I am naming her because I know she would want me to. I supported her sister Brenda to raise a complaint via PALS. What a complete waste of time that was. Rosie was an incredible person, she had more than her fair share of heartbreak in life, losing three of her four children in separate tragic instances, she also lost her husband, who tragically drowned whilst out fishing. On top of that she had numerous health issues to contend with, a number of strokes, the last one leaving her virtually blind. She also had kidney failure, all this ill health led to her numerous admissions to this ward over a number of years, and because of the way she was treated, she absolutely hated it. It was her worst nightmare, and tragically she died on that ward in the most cruel, cold and calculating way. We have kept all the documentation stating the catalogue of events prior to and leading up to her death. Including a development plan that was received in response to the complaint. It was from the ward manager, and unbelievably, one of the actions on this plan, was to remind qualified nurses of the need to act professionally at all times. I would like to remind them of the 5 Cs of caring, developed by Roach. Competence, Confidence, Commitment, Conscience and something that they absolutely should have been reminded of, Compassion, that Rosie most definitely was NOT shown. That along with a useless apology was the conclusion of the complaint. Oh, and did I mention the fact, she worked right up to her retirement, so was definitely not a drain on the system?

Sadly, there are lots of people I have spoken to who have similar tragic stories to this, and so this was not by far, an isolated case. Ironically, I was one of the many that stood and clapped for the NHS staff during the pandemic. Never again, I have lost all respect and feel very bitter towards them. Obviously, there are exceptions to this but in reality, not all are the caring angels of mercy we are led to believe. I have deliberately named the hospital and the ward, because I wanted to give Rosie a platform to be heard, however large or small it proves to be. Also, by naming them maybe it will trigger some kind of response, and give them something to reflect on, oh, I hope so. Legal advice was sought at the time, via the no win no fee route, but unfortunately, unless it is a very high percentage in favour of a win, for example a wrong leg being amputated, they won't take it on. However not one of them said it was unfounded, just that they couldn't help. The documents in their entirety are available if anyone in the legal profession is interested, or indeed if the staff on ward four wish to contest it, I say to them, "bring it on." Her sister Brenda and I would relish the opportunity to speak up publicly and for Rosie's voice to be heard from the grave.

Before I finish, I know Rosie would want me to mention the staff at the Kidney Dialysis Unit in North Tees Hospital Stockton. They were amazing, Rosie thought the absolute world of them, and they did her. They described her as the life and soul and were genuinely upset when she died, some of them even attended her funeral. What does that say about ward four, James Cook Hospital???

We have recently had a General Election on the 4th of July 2024. Not surprisingly, Labour have been voted in. Not the outcome I was hoping for, however I was willing to give them a chance. I was guessing at worst it would just be more of the same but OMG, no one could have predicted the behaviour of these self-serving politicians that we now have as our government. I could liken it to a comedy act, however that would make it funny, and funny it definitely is NOT. Anyway, no worries on that score, we only have the next five years of it to contend with, perish the thought.

Well, on that note, I really am going to end it there, I will leave you to your own views and opinions, that I think, at least for the time being, we are still just about entitled to voice.

As for me, I am now going to concentrate on living and enjoying the rest of my life, without worrying about any of the above. So, it's back to, head in the sand for me.

Que sera sera.

I hope you have enjoyed reading this book, as much as I have writing it.

Thank you, and best wishes to you all.

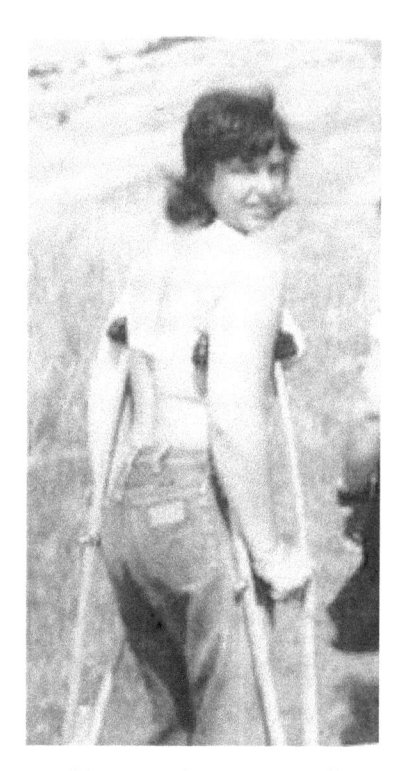

Me on a Country Walk   *Mam & Dad*

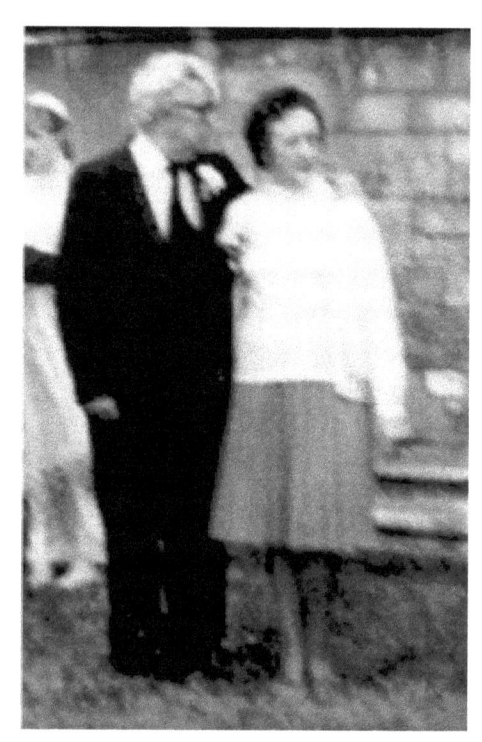

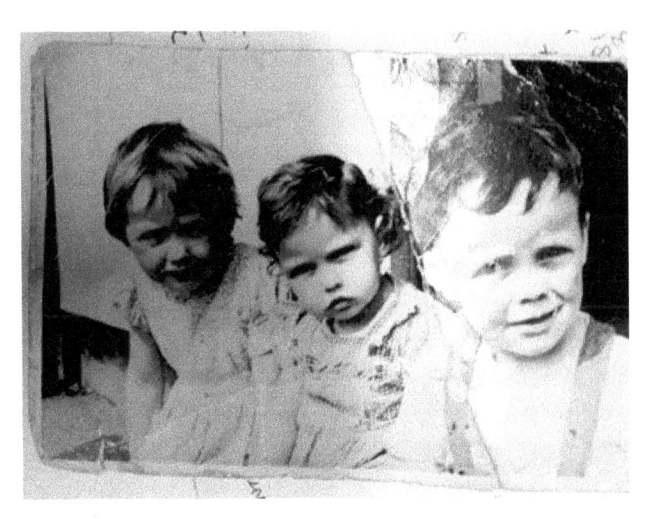

top whinging and just get on with it!!! My Life Growing up

Marjy, Myself & George

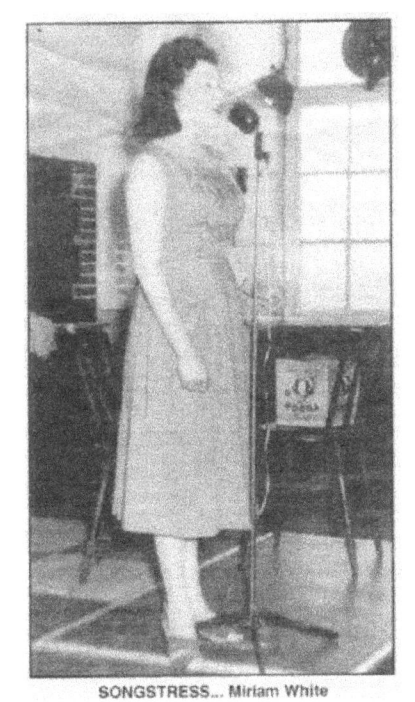

SONGSTRESS... Miriam White

Memories of a mellow maniac

Aunty Mim, my dad's sister, my claim to fame. Lol

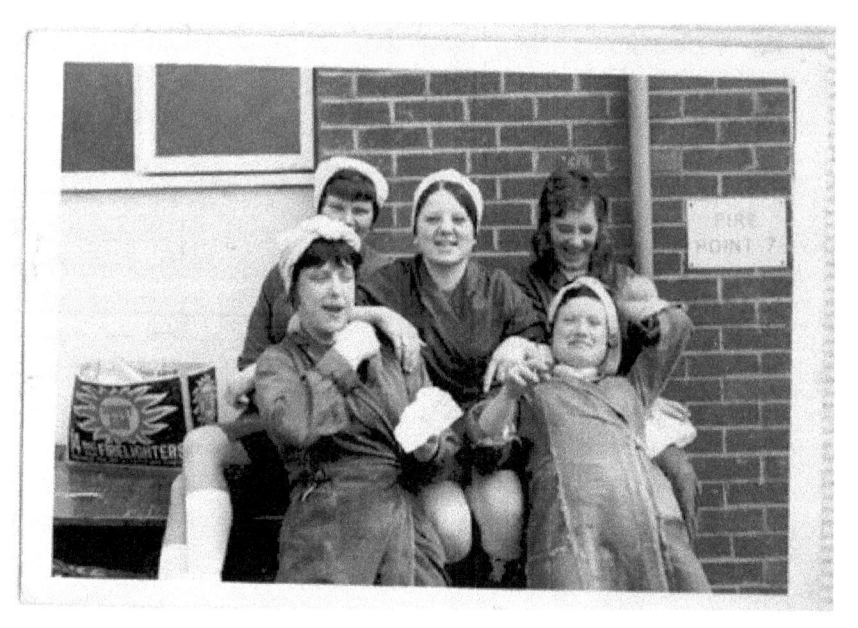

Happy Days at the Chicken Factory (Front Left, me)

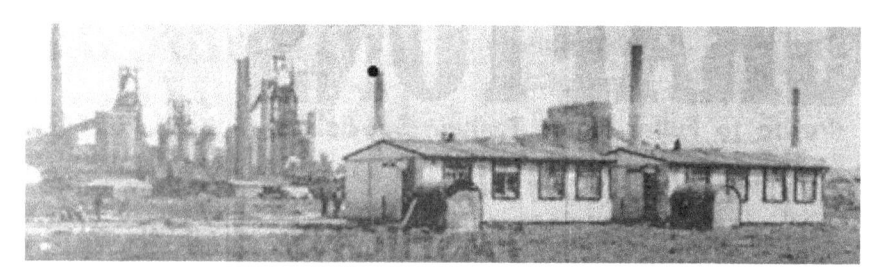

25 Bowness Grove, our first home

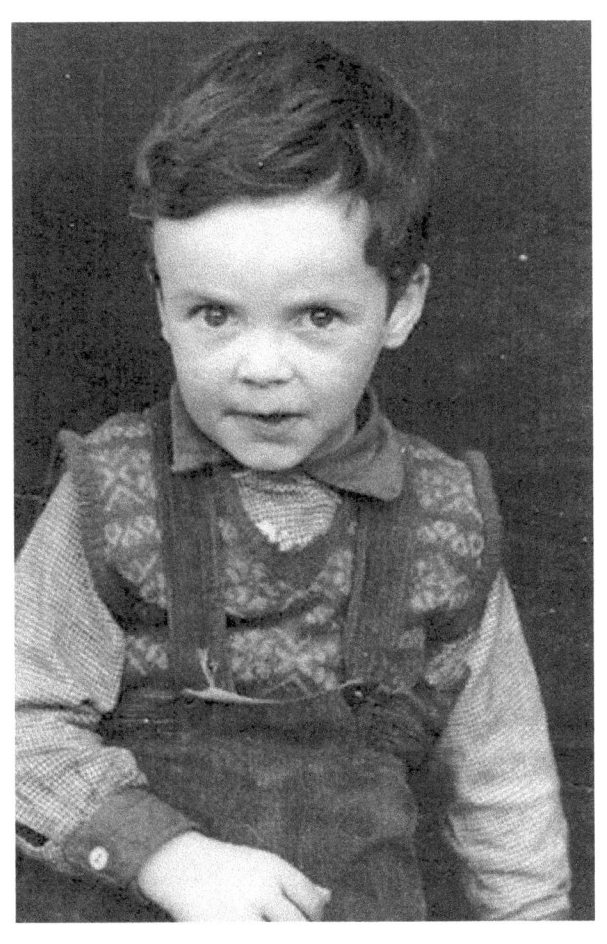

op whinging and just get on with it!!! My Life Growing up

My brother George bless him.

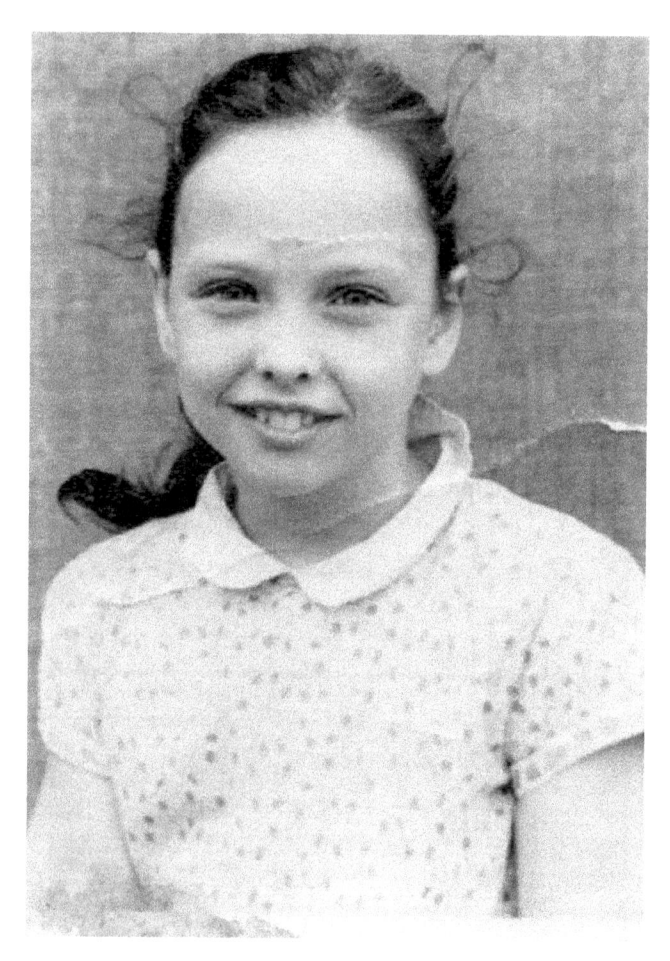

Me aged 9

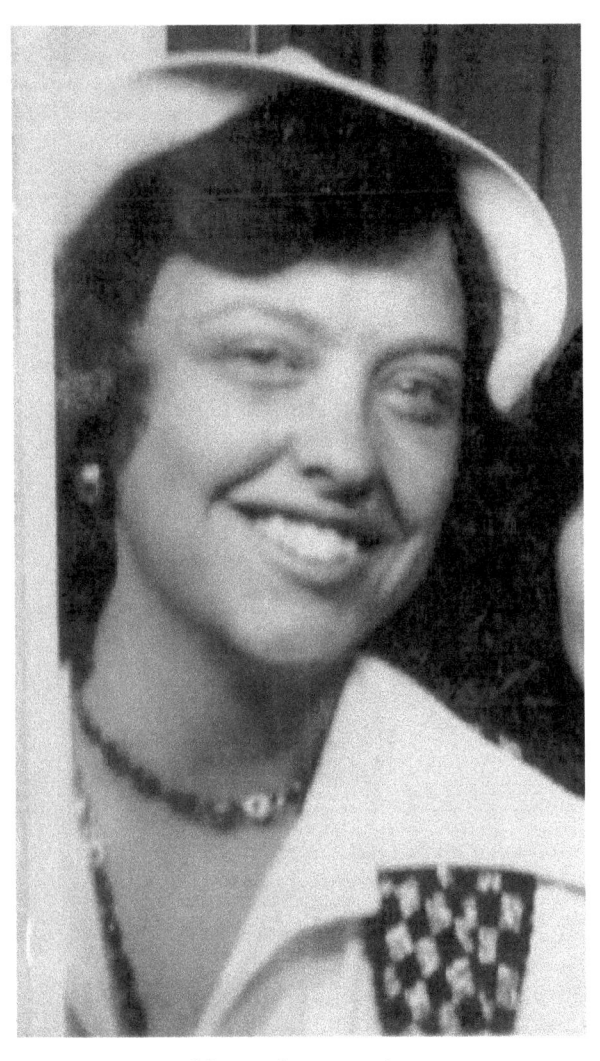

Me early twenties

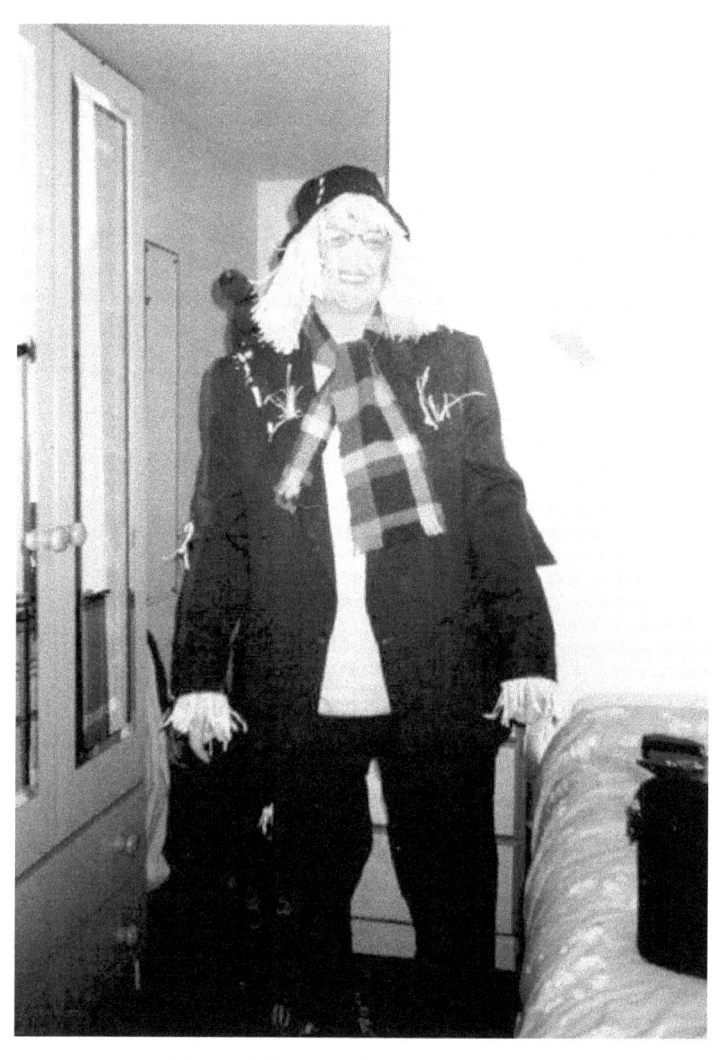

Worzel Gummidge Fancy Dress

My furry friends, past and present.

Penny "I'm coming with you" and she did lol. Penny was my first ever baby. What loyalty, I was her world and she mine, she passed at 18 years

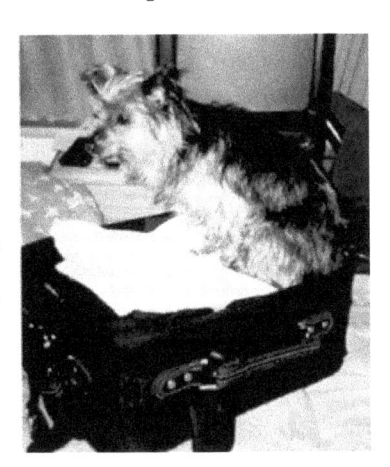

Tess. She was Penny's puppy and was tragically killed on the road aged two. Unfortunately, no photograph but a beautiful little girl she was.

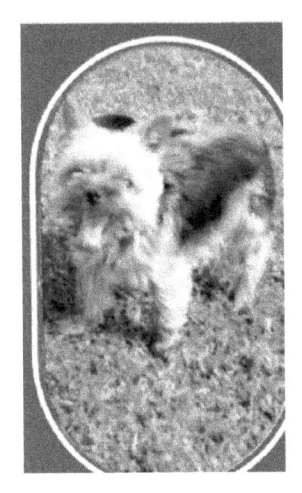

Cassie, was an amazing little doggie, throw a ball and she would run for miles. Sadly due, to veterinary neglect, she died aged nine.

Lilley, OMG she was amazing, the ramp was to help her onto her favourite chair, the cushions to break her fall, and yes, she couldn't always make it to the toilet, bless her. Recently passed aged, twenty-one.

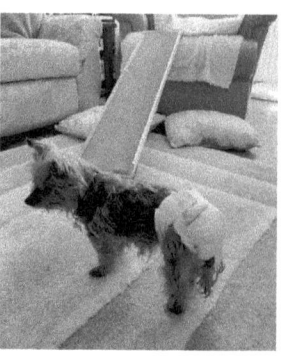

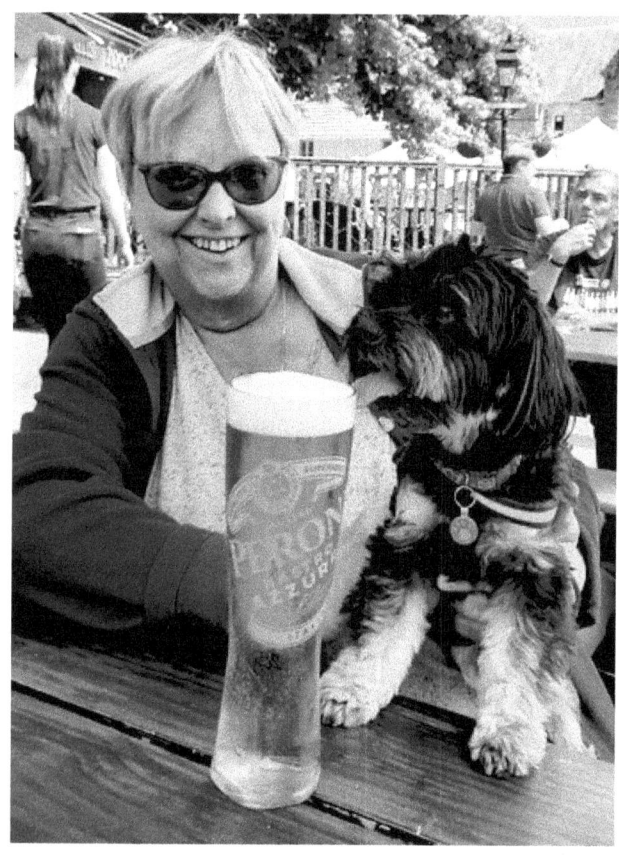

Dolly, is with me now, and like all my doggies she is amazing, currently 6 years old, here she is enjoying sharing my lager Lol.

Special thank you to my friend Swin Tempest for his support and for the amazing illustrations, a truly talented artist.

Also, a special thank you to my friend Jolene Brumby for her ongoing technical support, always ready to help, I couldn't have done it without you Jo.

Finally a big thank you to my family, all my friends, in fact to all the people who have touched my life in a positive way. You know who you are, I'm fortunate enough to say, there are too many to mention. I am truly blessed.

I'm enjoying the life I have chosen for myself, and I don't answer to anyone. So yes, in the main all in all, no regrets.

www.ingramcontent.com/pod-product-compliance
Ingram Content Group UK Ltd.
Pitfield, Milton Keynes, MK11 3LW, UK
UKHW030706160225
455163UK00013B/183